The Price of Pretty

Also by Alex Light

You Are Not a Before Picture:
How to Finally Make Peace with Your Body, for Good

The Price of Pretty

Alex Light

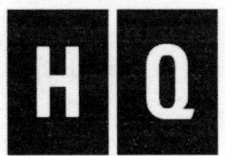

ONE PLACE. MANY STORIES

HQ
An imprint of HarperCollins*Publishers* Ltd
1 London Bridge Street
London SE1 9GF

www.harpercollins.co.uk

HarperCollins*Publishers*
Macken House, 39/40 Mayor Street Upper
Dublin 1, D01 C9W8, Ireland
This edition 2026

1
First published in Great Britain by HQ,
an imprint of HarperCollins*Publishers* Ltd 2026

Copyright © Alex Light 2026

Alex Light asserts the moral right to be identified as the author of this work.
A catalogue record for this book is available from the British Library.

HB ISBN: 978-0-00-871615-8
TPB ISBN: 978-0-00-871616-5

Set in Adobe Caslon Pro by HarperCollins*Publishers* India

All rights reserved. No part of this publication may be reproduced, stored
in a retrieval system, or transmitted, in any form or by any means,
electronic, mechanical, photocopying, recording or otherwise,
without the prior written permission of the publishers.

Without limiting the exclusive rights of any author, contributor or the publisher
of this publication, any unauthorised use of this publication to train generative
artificial intelligence (AI) technologies is expressly prohibited. HarperCollins also
exercise their rights under Article 4(3) of the Digital Single Market Directive 2019/790
and expressly reserve this publication from the text and data mining exception.

Printed and bound in the UK using 100% Renewable
Electricity at CPI Group (UK) Ltd

Contents

Introduction: How Did We End Up Back Here Again?   1

Chapter 1 Thin Is Back In   7
Chapter 2 The Ozempic Effect   43
Chapter 3 Family, Kids and Breaking the Cycle   71
Chapter 4 Pregnancy and Postpartum   103
Chapter 5 The 'Perfect' Face   130
Chapter 6 Make-Up   154
Chapter 7 The Tweakment Trap   173
Chapter 8 Over To You . . .   201

Conclusion   226
Acknowledgements   227
Endnotes   230

Introduction

How Did We End Up Back Here Again?

I chose to call my first book *You Are Not a Before Picture* because those five words felt like a revolution – one I wish I'd heard decades earlier. When I did hear them for the first time, it changed my life. For as long as I could remember, I'd thought of my body as something temporary – a 'before' version that I would eventually transform into an 'after'. As a result, I lived in a constant state of postponement: I'd go to the beach *after* I'd lost weight, I'd wear that cute dress *after* I'd 'toned' my arms, I'd be more confident, more desirable, just an all-round better version of myself . . . after.

Breaking free from that conditional way of living gave me permission to exist fully, in the present, in the body I was already in. It was liberating – it opened a door I didn't even know existed to body and mental peace. Of course, that peace didn't come easily – I had to unlearn decades of conditioning from growing up in the thin-obsessed 1990s and 2000s and the years spent absorbing calorie-counting magazine headlines, makeover shows and every single bit of messaging that told me I wasn't good enough. The work of untangling that mass of conditioning was slow and often painful – and heaven knows there were times when I just wanted to give up – but it was also the foundation of real freedom. And from there, I wanted to help other people to stop seeing themselves as projects, too. Far too many of us are living smaller lives than we deserve, holding ourselves back from joy, connection and opportunity until we feel like we have earned it through weight loss.

When I began writing *You Are Not a Before Picture* in 2022, it felt like we were on the precipice of a real cultural shift towards greater acceptance of more diverse representation. Brands were starting to cast bigger bodies in campaigns, the fashion industry was widening its size ranges at the demands of a now-emboldened consumer; and we were openly talking about diet culture in a way that felt brave and refreshing. It wasn't perfect, but there was undoubtedly a sense of momentum; of something changing.

I was aware that there was fragility in that progress – even in moments of celebration, the comment sections on plus-size campaigns were usually brutal, and there were whispers from corners of the internet and around dinner tables that maybe we'd 'gone too far' with all this 'body positivity'. The cracks were forming, but I truly had no idea how deep they would go – or how quickly everything could change again. These whispers were the first flickers of a backlash that I ignored in favour of trying to turn this newfound visibility into something permanent and lasting.

I wanted to open – and keep open – a conversation about the way we view our bodies; a conversation that challenged the relentless and ubiquitous pressure to shrink, tone, fix and perfect ourselves in pursuit of an ever-evolving beauty ideal. I wanted to expose the damage done by a culture that tells us we are always a work in progress, never quite good enough as we are.

I could never have anticipated the success of that book, both in terms of sales and, most importantly, in terms of reaction and reception. It resonated with so many people. The messages I received in response to the book, from those who told me they'd worn a swimsuit for the first time in years, eaten cake without guilt or finally appeared in photos with their children – are a gift I will cherish forever.

I poured everything I had into those pages. I cried sad tears, angry tears, happy tears and everything in between as I delved into my own relationship history with food and weight, and explored the devastating impact our diet culture-steeped society has on our body image. Writing that book was both liberating and exposing . . . I had to revisit old shame, name things I'd never said out loud and trust that honesty would connect me to others who felt the same. It was my most vulnerable work yet and I was so delighted – and, I must admit, relieved! – by the response.

Not too long after the book came out, though, I started to notice something unsettling. In the same feeds that had very recently been full of joyful, defiant posts that refused to conform to the ideals we'd long been held to, other trends were gaining momentum: videos began emerging that celebrated extreme thinness; 'glow-up' weight-loss transformations were appearing, alongside excited chatter about something called 'Ozempic', and a growing fixation with cosmetic 'tweaks'. Without really realizing it was happening, it felt as if the volume was slowly being turned down on body positivity, and cranked up on thinness, beauty 'discipline' and self-monitoring.

What I hadn't anticipated when I wrote *You Are Not a Before Picture*, was that there would be so, so much more to say; that body positivity and acceptance weren't done deals. At the time, it felt like we'd entered a new era, one free from the burden of thinness and instead defined by authenticity and embracing our softness. I truly thought – in hindsight, very naively – that we'd finally shifted the conversation for good.

But despite the strides made by the body positivity movement of the early 2020s, beauty standards made a sharp about-turn with the rise of weight-loss drugs, and thin is undeniably back in: catwalk models are as thin as they ever were, red carpets are arguably thinner, brands have shrunk back their size offerings and social media is once again preoccupied with being 'skinny'.

Weight-loss drugs promising rapid and dramatic transformations – at a price, of course, and we'll get into that – are being marketed to women as a solution to a problem we were never meant to have in the first place. What's more, filters are no longer just a playful addition to a selfie – they have become a prerequisite for presenting ourselves to the world. Cosmetic tweaks like Botox, filler and plastic surgery – once reserved for celebrities and the super-rich – are now as routine as getting your hair done.

I have spent years navigating this world, both personally and professionally. I have been on the receiving end of these impossible beauty standards, and I know first-hand how deeply they can shape a person's self-worth. As someone who has struggled with body image and disordered eating, I understand the emotional weight of these pressures. My work has also taken me beyond my own experience. I've spent years researching the subject, interviewing experts to better inform myself, and engaging in honest conversations with thousands of women who feel much the same way as I do. As you peel back the layers of the beauty myth and unpack it, you can't help but start to question – who is it that is benefiting from all of this? And at what cost to the rest of us?

That's why I felt I had to write this book. It feels like we are at a tipping point. The beauty standards we face today have become increasingly unattainable: we're not just being asked to be thin anymore, but also sculpted, smooth, eternally youthful and filtered to perfection. These expectations continue to escalate, and the stakes are getting higher. The financial cost, the emotional toll and even the risks to our physical health are mounting. So, this book is my deep dive into the world we are living in right now, particularly as women. I want to examine the forces shaping today's beauty ideals, the rise of new technologies and treatments, and the industries profiting from our insecurities.

Just as importantly, I want to continue the conversation about self-acceptance; about reclaiming our bodies from the endless cycle of 'fixing' and 'improving'. If we don't continue questioning those pressures, we will stay stuck in an eternal loop, endlessly chasing an impossible standard – and should we really let that be our reality?

I hope this book helps us see things more clearly. I hope it sparks conversations that lead to real change. And most of all,

I hope it reminds you that *you* were never the problem in the first place.

At the end of each chapter that follows, you'll find a few questions to help you reflect on what you've read, and to think about how each topic is impacting you in your own life. They can be used as journaling prompts, or they may spark a new train of thought. I hope you find them useful.

Chapter 1

Thin Is Back In

It pains me to say it, but the stark and undeniable truth is this: body positivity is dead and thin is back in.

Scroll through your Instagram or TikTok feed and it's hard to miss – we've returned to a world in which protruding hip bones, concave stomachs and pin-thin limbs are framed as aspirational once again. 'Thin' appears to be the ultimate, and only, standard of beauty. Of course, thinness never really left; it has underpinned our culture for decades. But something about its current resurgence feels sharper and more unapologetic than before. On TikTok, it even has its own corner of the internet: #SkinnyTok; a subculture where videos romanticising extreme thinness are curated and served to users – primarily, young women and girls. It's horrifying and, honestly, almost unbelievable how explicit some of this content is: 'body check' videos of very thin women with taglines like 'being skinny is an outfit'; 'advice' videos on how to 'be a skinny legend' (spoiler: restriction is key); and 'tough love' videos that attempt to shame viewers into not eating ('You need a treat? WTF are you – a dog?'). Other posts are more subtle, with the underlying diet culture hidden behind pastel filters, 'wellness' language and 'what I eat in a day' videos that happen to skip breakfast and mainly comprise of low-calorie, low-carb foods, making them harder to spot but still hugely damaging.

In many ways, this era echoes the culture of the early 2000s and 'pro-ana' content (which promotes anorexia), but it has a shinier, slightly more socially acceptable veneer – and, worryingly, it seems to be more mainstream than pro-ana content ever was. Back in the early-2000s, the blogging and social media site Tumblr was used by some as an underground network for disordered eating and eating disorders, where users shared 'thinspiration' photos of emaciated models and endless 'motivational' quotes; traded tips on how best to suppress hunger; and romanticised hospital wristbands as proof of 'dedication' to being thin. It was tucked away from the mainstream, and that secrecy was part of its danger. When I was unwell, I found pockets of the internet that fuelled my eating disorders and validated my most harmful behaviours, but it wasn't easy to find. The only real access to pro-ana content I had was via Tumblr, and I had to search for it. Now, unfortunately, that kind of content finds you. You don't have to look for it: the precision-engineered algorithm serves it up the moment you engage with a post about weight, food or fitness – or even if you don't! Simply being profiled as a girl or a woman is enough for social media platforms to push, or at least suggest, this type of content – particularly given that social media is so saturated with it right now.

The most terrifying part is that this kind of content is rewarded by the platforms through reach, engagement and visibility. An algorithm doesn't know the difference between what's helpful or harmful, it just knows that certain content keeps people watching, and for someone in the grips of an eating disorder, that feedback loop – watch, get shown more, watch again – can be extremely dangerous and addictive, reinforcing and normalizing unhealthy beliefs and behaviours. Given the pervasiveness of this content, it can be incredibly difficult to escape, and therefore incredibly hard to protect yourself from – and I say this as a 36-year-old woman who has had years of therapy, and who lives and breathes rejecting diet culture. If I find it hard to avoid, then what chance does a vulnerable teenager have?

Part of the problem is the sheer speed and scale at which these ideals now spread. Because of their powerful algorithms, trends on platforms like TikTok or Instagram travel at lightning speed, reaching millions of people in hours. Cultural shifts in aesthetic ideals crash into our feeds before we've even caught our breath from the last one. Unlike previous eras of glossy magazines and fashion exclusivity, this new wave of thinness isn't just presented to us through models and celebrities: it's reinforced by influencers and 'real people' whose lives we get to peer into daily via social media. It's no longer just a photoshoot in *Vogue* or a billboard in Times Square; it's a friend at the gym posting mirror selfies with captions about 'discipline' or a viral 'before and after' video featuring drastic weight loss framed as a 'glow-up'. This is also what makes it so insidious: it slips into our personal spaces. And because it often comes from people we 'know' – friends, friends of friends, co-workers, classmates – it feels less like marketing and more like . . . just a fact of life? The technology we interact with constantly invites, or rather, demands comparison.

The rise of powerful new weight-loss drugs has poured petrol on the fire. GLP-1 medications like Ozempic, Wegovy and Mounjaro, originally developed as a treatment for diabetes, have supercharged the conversation and arguably fast-tracked the trend of thinness, making weight loss look both desirable and now *effortless*. You can see the ripple effects everywhere: celebrities are shrinking; influencers are euphemising their transformations with phrases like 'getting healthy'; and fashion brands that once embraced body diversity are quietly retreating back to sample sizes and ultra-thin silhouettes. It's a far cry from where we were just a few years ago.

The Power of Body Positivity

Before it became a social media slogan, body positivity began as a radical act of resistance. The movement's roots reach back to the fat liberation activism of the 1960s and 1970s – a campaign grounded in social justice, equality and the visibility of fat bodies. Early activists fought against systemic discrimination in healthcare, employment and media representation. Their aim wasn't to inspire confidence or self-love necessarily; it was to demand dignity. As the movement grew, Black feminists and queer activists deepened its politics, connecting body liberation to broader struggles against racism, sexism and heteronormativity.

Over time, those radical roots were absorbed into mainstream culture. As the language of 'body positivity' spread through social media, its focus largely shifted from collective liberation to personal empowerment.

Fast forward to 2014, when underwear company Aerie announced it would cease airbrushing its imagery, launching the

#AerieREAL campaign, which aimed to celebrate women 'as they are'. Featuring plus-size model Iskra Lawrence, who became the ambassador for the brand, this was one of the first 'body positive' campaigns I had ever been exposed to, and its impact left me truly dumbstruck. Never before had I seen a brand – and an underwear brand no less! – showcase bodies that looked even remotely like mine, with soft stomachs, hip dips, flaws and all. I wanted to print the campaign images out, frame them and hang them in every room in my house. I wanted to set it as the wallpaper on my home screen. A touch dramatic? Maybe, but it meant a lot to me, and to other women too. These weren't the perfectly polished, impossibly toned bodies we'd been conditioned to associate with beauty or desirability; they were real, relatable – and crucially, they were not part of a transformation story. These bodies weren't a 'before' photo – they were being celebrated exactly as they were. It felt like a direct challenge to everything I had grown up believing about what women were 'supposed' to look like, and I distinctly remember having the feeling – because I don't think it was a conscious, concrete thought but more of a sentiment at that time – that maybe there wasn't actually anything wrong with my body. I was still years away from really, truly believing that, but I know without doubt that it planted a seed.

I gasped when I saw plus-size model Tess Holliday gracing the cover of *Cosmopolitan* in 2018. Wearing an emerald-green satin swimsuit and blowing a kiss to the camera, the plus-size model unapologetically showed off her fat body in an act of defiance that challenged decades of oppressive beauty standards. The cover ignited a cultural firestorm – it was hailed as a victory for body positivity by some and condemned as 'glorifying obesity' by others.

But naysayers and critics aside, it felt like a seminal moment: it unleashed a sense of hope that the world was finally ready to embrace a more inclusive definition of beauty and provide us with greater visibility of bodies that had previously been pushed to the margins of society.

Widely considered the poster girl of modern-day body positivity, plus-size model Ashley Graham broke lots of new ground in the body image space in the late 2010s: having made history by becoming the first curvy model to grace the cover of the *Sports Illustrated Swimsuit* in 2016, she was also the first ever plus-size model to appear on the cover of revered fashion bible *British Vogue* in 2017, a fashion magazine renowned for its glorification of thinness. It's worth noting that she featured alongside six other, straight-size models, with her body barely visible, but it was *Vogue*'s first step into plus-size territory and consequently, it was a very big deal. It was in 2019 that Ashley really helped flip social media beauty standards on its head, however: one of her most notable posts featured an intimate close-up of her body – the type of body that felt familiar to so many of us, yet one that, as women, we'd been taught to fear and fix. The photo amassed almost 1.4 million likes and over 24,000 comments, most of which were women praising Ashley and thanking her for making them feel more 'normal'. The surge of appreciation was indicative of the appetite for this kind of 'relatable' content, and a stream of influencers – me included – followed suit, sharing our own 'authentic' images online.

At this point in my life, I felt like I was coming out of the other side of my eating disorder and felt incredibly motivated to kick my demons to the kerb once and for all. Sharing pictures of my body seemed like a great way to throw myself into the deep end, as well as helping others who might be struggling to feel perhaps just a little better about their own bodies. I posted a series of photos of my body unposed, showing stretch marks, cellulite, rolls and images that were typically 'unflattering', with #bodypositive quotes laid over the top, encouraging people to tap into their own self-love. It was incredibly scary at first to be so vulnerable – exposing the parts of myself I'd spent years trying to hide felt like peeling back layers I wasn't sure I was ready to shed. But the response was overwhelming: messages poured in from people who said they finally felt seen, or that for the first time in a long time, they felt like their body wasn't 'wrong'. It made me realize just how starved we all were for realness – raw, vulnerable, imperfect authenticity. What started as a deeply personal protest against the private, personal shame that I'd carried for so long quickly became a collective experience; part of something so much bigger than just me and my camera roll. It was a digital rebellion; a mass unlearning of everything we'd internalized from years of toxic messaging.

With each picture of a woman whose body looked like ours, or like our mum, our sister or our friend, it felt like we were all finally exhaling, releasing a lifetime's worth of suffocating pressure to be perfect. We'd been holding our breath without even realizing it.

Research backs this up, too: a 2023 study[1] showed that following social media pages celebrating different body shapes, sizes, colours and abilities can help improve young women's body image in everyday life. Researchers from the School of Psychology, UNSW Science, found that women aged 18-25 who viewed body positive posts daily over a 14-day period reported a decrease in body dissatisfaction and less tendency to compare their appearance online with others. Their improvements in body image were also maintained four weeks after viewing the content. The lead author of the study, Dr Jasmine Fardouly, concluded: 'A very brief intervention over a short time where young women viewed a small number of body-positive posts among the social media content they're regularly viewing was able to improve body image and reduce body comparisons.' This wasn't an isolated finding either. A 2024 study[2] found that simply showing participants body-positive imagery improved body satisfaction and reduced the drive to conform to thin ideals in both men and women. Another study found that seeing images of diverse bodies increased body compassion.[3] For many participants, the effect was almost immediate: seeing people who looked like them, or like someone they loved, seemed to create an instant recalibration of what a 'normal' body looks like.

We also know that representation can shift the baseline of how we think about our bodies altogether: research on body diversity in reality TV, for example, found that viewers exposed to a wider range of body types reported higher self-esteem and a stronger sense of belonging.[4] The common thread in all this evidence is simple but profound: representation and body diversity matter. We need to see bodies that look like ours reflected back at us, and when we do, it loosens the grip of the impossible ideal and offers us hope that there is more than one way to have a 'good' body. All this research validated what I'd been seeing in my own work. For a while, it felt like we were genuinely rewriting the rules of beauty and creating a world where more people were going to be allowed to just exist without apology.

Backlash

For all this progress that seemed to be happening, it's worth noting that any wins in terms of body positivity in the media were always met with pushback. As already mentioned, Tess Holliday's cover feature in *Cosmopolitan* was *really* divisive, sparking worldwide debate that mostly revolved around Tess's health. Of course, Tess's health was nobody else's business but her own, but that didn't stop the likes of Piers Morgan using his slot on morning television to debate it at length. A similar pattern played out again in 2019 when Nike introduced a plus-size mannequin into its flagship London store. This was undoubtedly a positive step for body diversity, but wow! was it controversial: the brand's move became a nationwide talking point and we were inundated with think-pieces about how our society was enabling and 'promoting obesity'. 'Obese mannequins are selling a dangerous lie', ran a headline in the *Telegraph*.

The backlash completely missed the point – as it so often does. This wasn't about glorifying anything; it was about representation. It was about someone walking into a shop and, maybe for the first time in their life, seeing a body that looked like theirs in a space traditionally reserved for the thin and athletic. It was about making movement and exercise feel accessible and welcoming to *everyone*, not just people in smaller bodies. And yet, somehow, the conversation was hijacked and twisted into another tired debate about health, with outrage fuelled not by concern, let's be honest here, but instead by the deep-rooted discomfort our culture has around fatness. What should have been a moment of progress – one of inclusion and visibility – became yet another reminder of just how far we still had to go. It also perfectly illustrates the double bind that people in bigger bodies face: they're relentlessly told to lose weight, exercise, take responsibility for their health – and yet, when they *do* engage in movement, or when they appear in activewear campaigns, they're met with outrage. It's hard not to feel as if you're damned if you do, damned if you don't.

At the risk of labouring the point about the backlash towards body positivity, we can't talk about body diversity in the public eye without covering the rise of plus-size singer, Lizzo. She skyrocketed to fame in 2016 for her empowering lyrics that were full of affirmations like 'thick thighs save lives' and 'feeling good as hell', which cemented her as a body positivity icon. The image of the star strutting around the Glastonbury stage in a skin-tight holographic purple leotard playing a flute will be forever etched into my memory. But Lizzo's newfound icon status brought with it an army of naysayers, desperate to share their personal views and opinion on her health. Fitness media personality Jillian Michaels, trainer on the US weight-loss show *The Biggest Loser*, discussed Lizzo's appearance in 2020 after being asked why people were 'celebrating' the musician's body. 'Why does it matter?' she said. 'Why aren't we celebrating her music? Cause it isn't going to be awesome if she gets diabetes.' This kind of commentary reveals so much about, again, the double standard that fat people are held to, and how society so often dresses up its prejudice as 'concern'. There's no way that, had Lizzo been thin, anyone would have asked Jillian Michaels to comment on her body at all. The conversation wouldn't have been about health; it would have been about her talent or her performance. But because Lizzo exists in a larger body, her health is suddenly treated as fair game, and her body is treated like a public problem in need of correction. This health argument, so often trotted out as concern when it comes to people living in bigger bodies, is anything but genuine. We don't tend to interrogate the health of thin celebrities who drink excessively, under-eat, over-exercise or party non-stop because, crucially, their bodies conform to the ideal. We demand that fat people both justify their existence through the lens of health and perform health to us – and even then, it's not enough.

Lizzo's popularity, it's worth noting, took a sharp downturn in 2023 when the singer was hit by a string of allegations, including sexual harassment and fostering a hostile work environment, filed by three former backup dancers. Lizzo denied these allegations, describing them as 'unbelievable' and 'too outrageous not to be addressed'. But the lawsuits had a significant impact on her career, leading to cancelled performances and lost sponsorships. In 2024, Lizzo announced on Instagram that she was 'quitting' and it's important to note that in her statement about leaving, she cited part of the reason was 'being the butt of the joke every single time because of how I look'. In 2025, she made a much-embraced return.

It's impossible to ignore the fact that Lizzo has lost a significant amount of weight in recent years. She's spoken about it at length on her Instagram and TikTok, framing it as part of a broader journey towards health, strength and balance. For many of her fans – particularly plus-size women who had seen Lizzo as living proof that you could exist joyfully and unapologetically and be hugely successful in a fat body – the change was a tough pill to swallow. Some felt disappointed, even betrayed. When the world is so reluctant to spotlight and celebrate plus-size people, losing one can feel personal. For years, Lizzo had represented hope and possibility to many, and her weight loss reminded them how fragile and conditional that representation can be. But honestly, can we blame Lizzo for losing weight? After years of being dissected, mocked and often reduced to nothing more than a debate about whether or not her body was acceptable or healthy, is it any wonder that she might want to move through the world with a little less of that relentless scrutiny? Of course, I can't know for certain her motivations for losing weight, but I'd love it if we could give her the benefit of the doubt, because I'd challenge anyone not to be ground down by the level of vitriol she has endured, and continues to endure. We're quick to tell women to ignore the haters, to rise above it and be strong, but the truth is that existing in a fat body in public, let alone on the world stage, is tough, and sometimes the easiest thing to do isn't refusing to change but to make the changes you need to simply survive.

It is another illustration of the impossible double bind women are constantly placed in. When we gain weight, we're accused of 'letting ourselves go' and being 'unhealthy', and when we lose it, we're accused of betraying the cause.

Tangible Changes

Despite all the backlash, it seemed evident that body positivity had finally become mainstream and the needle was being moved in the right direction – and that alone was worthy of celebration, because bigger bodies were *finally* being allowed to take up just a fraction of the spotlight, and any representation in the media of those who exist outside of the beauty standard is huge. This, along with viral posts like Ashley Graham's that unapologetically showcased familiar, relatable bodies that weren't filtered or airbrushed to perfection, helped to normalize what had long been deemed unacceptable. Suddenly, our social media feeds were sprinkled with unposed angles and reminders that fat wasn't a 'flaw'. It was a direct contrast to the flawless, impossibly thin women who filled the pages of the magazines we pored over as children and teenagers. Finally, the narrative was changing. The self-acceptance, inclusion and diversity messages of this iteration of body positivity brought with it more than just a shift in print media and social media. For as long as capitalism has existed and for as long as diet culture has been a defining force in our everyday lives, it has felt like we have been at the mercy of brands and marketeers, powerless against the narratives pushed on us in advertising. But with the rise of the body positivity movement, it was clear that public appetite had changed, and companies were forced to pivot on their usual, surefire ways of making money and bringing in customers.

Brands began expanding their size ranges and casting models in a wider range of sizes to advertise their clothes and products. Fashion and beauty campaigns suddenly centred around diversity: for the first time, we saw unretouched skin with visible stretch marks, tummy rolls, body hair, and bodies that didn't fit the narrow mould we'd been force-fed for so long. Brands like Aerie, ASOS, Dove and Savage X Fenty made headlines by showing models of varying shapes, size, races, abilities and genders.

More model diversity was suddenly not only expected but demanded on the catwalks – even designer catwalks, believe it or not. Ashley Graham walked for Dolce & Gabbana in 2018 and Fendi in 2020; fashion brands were called on to expand their size ranges, and companies were challenged to evolve in ways they *never* had before. In the Spring/Summer 2020 season, 86 plus-size models walked runways across all four major cities – this accounted for 2.8 per cent of all models. That figure may sound pitiful, but in the context of an industry like fashion, which has historically excluded fat bodies altogether, it was a meaningful shift. It felt like designers were beginning to acknowledge that fashion shouldn't be reserved for one body type. It was a long way from perfect, but it was a definite step toward visibility, inclusion and undoing the damage of decades of erasure.

The shift felt even more significant given the cultural context we were emerging from: the thin-obsessed era of the late 1990s and early 2000s. This was the age of heroin chic, low-rise jeans and the peak of tabloid body-shaming – a time when women's bodies were relentlessly picked apart in the media. Paparazzi photos of female celebrities were splashed across magazine covers with headlines like 'Baby Bump or Just Bloated?' or 'She's Let Herself Go!'. The ideal body type – impossibly thin, white, toned but crucially not *too* muscular – was upheld as the standard that everyone should aspire to. It was a particularly toxic time in history for body image, and one that left deep scars for a lot of us. By contrast, the late 2010s offered a glimmer of something different and *so* hopeful. For the first time in mainstream memory, there was space – though arguably, it was limited and still imperfect – for bodies that had been long invisible and pushed to the margins of society.

The most famous example of this is Weight Watchers. Amid a landscape that was increasingly wary of diet culture, in 2018, Weight Watchers changed its name to WW, two letters now attached to the tagline 'Wellness That Works' to distance itself from overt branding around dieting. The cereal Special K also attempted to shift its image from dieting to empowerment. Formerly well-known for its diet plan that encouraged replacing meals with bowls of cereal and cereal bars to lose weight, in 2017, it released an advert highlighting women's achievements whilst subtly connecting to the act of eating. 'Women are amazing. Our bodies grow babies. We run marathons, companies, solve problems. We eat,' the ad proclaimed. The campaign received mixed reactions, perhaps unsurprisingly: it was clunky at best, oversimplifying feminist messages and awkwardly linking them to the act of eating . . . cereal.

Most 'positive' shifts made by brands were, let's face it, pretty transparently shallow, and often felt forced. Slapping slogans about self-love onto campaigns and including a plus-size model in one ad didn't erase decades of exclusive and harmful messaging. The gestures often felt like quick PR fixes rather than meaningful commitments to change. Lane Byrant, the US clothing brand, which focuses on plus-size women, released its #I'mNoAngel campaign in 2015 as a response to Victoria's Secret's glorification of ultra-thin, conventionally attractive models they labelled 'angels' (we'll come back to them, don't worry). The Lane Bryant campaign aimed to challenge narrow beauty ideals by celebrating plus-size bodies, but it was soon called out for only showcasing a very specific type of 'curvy': hourglass figures with fairly flat stomachs, with all six of the models appearing to be quite similar in terms of size. It felt more like a curated response than a true embrace of body diversity, highlighting that even 'inclusive' representation can be very narrow.

Real-World Impacts

It's worth interrogating, at this point, how actual, real women were feeling during this period. Did this apparent cultural shift translate into real changes in how we saw ourselves, or were we still stuck in the same cycles of shame and comparison, just with a few more body types appearing on our Instagram feeds? It's a difficult question to answer. Body image isn't easily measured, and while there are studies on media representation and self-esteem, there is limited comprehensive, long-term data on how the body positivity movement affected the average woman. Instead, I'll speak to what I've observed, both within my own community and in the countless conversations I've had with women over the years. I know that, despite the glossy campaigns and empowering '#LoveYourself' hashtags, many women still felt like their bodies weren't the *right* kind of different. They didn't see themselves in the curated, polished and palatable version of body positivity that was gaining traction online, where plus-size models still had flat stomachs, chiselled jawlines and hourglass curves. For some, the body positivity movement became yet another impossible standard – a new kind of perfection to fall short of. If you didn't love your body loudly and unapologetically, if you struggled with acceptance, and if you still felt insecure or uncomfortable in your own skin, were you failing at empowerment, too? I think the reality is that a lot of women felt caught between two conflicting messages: on the one hand, society still implicitly demanded that they shrink themselves, and on the other, there was also an expectation that women celebrate the very bodies they'd been taught to despise all their lives. It was a kind of emotional whiplash that felt heavy and difficult to navigate for many. That said, it's undeniable that seeing a bigger variety of bodies celebrated in mainstream spaces had a positive impact. For many, especially those who had never seen themselves reflected in media before, or who didn't believe that their body type would ever have the right to be celebrated, it offered a crucial moment of recognition.

However imperfectly they were delivered and received, those moments of visibility planted important seeds. They gave language to experiences and ideas that we didn't even know existed, never mind knew how to articulate. They introduced concepts like fatphobia, diet culture and body autonomy into the public discourse in ways that hadn't existed before, and they made it easier – and more socially acceptable – to reject harmful norms, unfollow toxic accounts and question the need to shrink ourselves at all costs. In the many conversations I've had over the years about body image, I've heard countless women describe the positive effect that the body positivity movement had on their self-esteem. I've heard many refer to that period as a 'relief', while others have said that it was the first time they truly understood that the problem was never with their body, but rather with the world that had taught them to hate it.

Reversing Positivity

Now look: most of us are reluctant to think back to 2020, because it wasn't the greatest time in the world by any means, but it did play a vitally important part in the timeline of the body positivity movement. Along with unprecedented levels of stress, anxiety and depression, the onset of the quarantine restrictions prompted a huge uptick in social media consumption. Essentially, we were spending all day, every day on our phones, seeking the connection that had been lost as a result of the lockdowns. While there was some weight- and body-related pressure on social media during this time – you might remember people talking about the Quarantine15, referring to 15 lb of weight gain one might observe due to the mandates to stay indoors – there was a parallel stream of body positive content, and the trend of people sharing their authentic, unretouched and unposed pictures really underwent a meteoric rise in this period. No matter what their account had centred around previously, most influencers took part in this trend in one way or another: it felt like Instagram had exploded with authentic, real depictions of bodies and it was an enormous contrast to the glossy, curated Instagram we were so familiar with.

What I didn't realize at the time, though, in the midst of this wave of body positivity, is that even the most powerful movements can lose momentum – and the body positivity movement was no exception. Because the movement, whether we call it self-love or body positivity, was a trend, and as with all trends, they come and go. The #bodypositivity hashtag gradually lost momentum and we witnessed a slow and subtle but definite shift as the authentic images gradually became replaced once again with the flawless, glossy squares we had previously associated with Instagram. Public backlash against body diversity entered new territory, with more and more people loudly voicing their objections to the movement. Some influencers did an about-turn and deemed the idea of being body positive a 'lie', while some Instagram users took to the app to explain how consuming body positive content had led to weight gain. The conversation around the link between health and weight seemed to take on a new life: you couldn't scroll for more than two minutes without discovering a zealous rant from a man with a microphone declaring that we were all going to die instantly if our BMI went over 25.

The pandemic took a stark toll on our body image, too. The sudden rise of online meetings and constant video calls meant we were confronted with our own faces and bodies more than ever before. Every perceived flaw was staring back at us in real time, and by the time lockdowns lifted, the cultural pressure for a so-called 'hot girl summer' was in full swing, fuelling a renewed fixation on dieting, 'toning up' and looking 'better' than we did in isolation.

Just like that, the body positivity era seemed to be dying in front of our very eyes. Brands were just as quick to jump off the body diversity bandwagon as they were to jump on and the fashion industry, a space historically riddled with fatphobia and the unashamed glorification of thinness, was suspiciously eager to lean back into the thin ideal. After several years of breaking new ground by showcasing plus-size models on the runways during fashion weeks and extending clothing sizes (all of which honestly feels pathetic to even write), the focus on accommodating anyone above a size 8 was downgraded as a priority and people living in larger bodies once again found themselves lacking the representation they deserve.

The Kardashians, meanwhile, known for spearheading the 'slim-thick' trend of the 2010s – flat stomachs, tiny waists and wide hips and bum – noticeably slimmed down. They were even reported to have reversed their Brazilian Butt Lifts – a surgery in which fat is taken from the waist and injected into the bum. It's also one of the deadliest cosmetic procedures: in 2018, the American Society of Plastic Surgeons estimated that the death rate for those undergoing the surgery was 1 in 3,000. The 'slim-thick' look had been one of the defining beauty ideals of the late 2010s, but it's important to acknowledge that this body ideal was not new: the exaggerated curves that became 'fashionable' under the Kardashians' influence were rooted in a body type historically associated with Black women. For decades, these same features had been hypersexualised, mocked or used as a justification to dehumanise Black women in media. Yet, when light-skinned women with access to the world's best surgeons adopted a curated, surgically enhanced version of these features, they were suddenly reframed as aspirational. Now, just as quickly as it was popularised, the trend had shifted again. The BBL look fell out of favour and the Kardashians' visibly slimmer frames were celebrated by the tabloids.

The Return to Thinness

At the end of 2022, the *New York Post* published a headline declaring 'heroin chic is back', using the same trend-focused language that we would apply to a new pair of jeans to refer to our actual, physical bodies. Although the publication copped a tonne of backlash for the article, it seemed to be the final nail in the coffin for body diversity in the media and, in turn of course, our cultural acceptance of it. This societal shift coincided with the FDA's approval of semaglutide or GLP-1 for weight loss – and it's safe to say it was a perfect storm. Any progress or wins that we might have made seemed to have been wiped out with the arrival of this shiny new needle promising rapid weight loss.

Thinness in Hollywood is nothing new. It's been the default for as long as the industry has existed – you could almost call it a prerequisite for entry to the inner circle of La La Land. In 2023, however, a new, sharper iteration emerged on the red carpet: ultra-thin. It was now less about simply fitting into sample sizes and more about jutting collarbones and gowns that hung from tiny frames. The American Society of Plastic Surgeons dubbed the 'ballet body' as a new beauty trend, which should perhaps have prompted some concern. Ballet has long been notorious for its obsession with uniformity: it's an art form that prizes slenderness, symmetry and restraint. The world over, dancers are taught from childhood to make themselves smaller and lighter, and the ideal body in the ballet world is one so slender that it almost looks weightless, disciplined to the point of disappearance. When beauty culture starts suggesting that we should all draw inspiration from the harsh and disciplined world of ballet, it feels somewhat insidious.

In 2024, Victoria's Secret made an . . . interesting return to its famous catwalk show. Since its inception, Victoria's Secret has built a reputation on one principle: a narrow, impeccably flawless standard of beauty. The annual fashion show was much more than just a lingerie showcase – it was a cultural phenomenon, attracting millions of viewers each year. At its peak, the 2011 broadcast had a production budget nearing $12 million, and yet inclusion and diversity were all but invisible. Beyond the dazzling spectacle of pink feathers and diamantes, the backstage narratives revealed the true cost of achieving that standard: the *Guardian* alleged a grim underbelly in 2018, describing extreme diets, obsessive training and no plus-size models, warning that the beauty standards of Victoria's Secret models were a 'dangerous fantasy'. Model testimonies reinforced this problematic nature: in a stark confession, former angel Erin Heatherton revealed in 2021 that she resorted to phentermine (an appetite suppressant) and HCG injections. HCG stands for human chorionic gonadotropin; a hormone made during pregnancy. Primarily used to treat infertility, the drug has also been used, incorrectly, for weight loss, despite not being approved for the purpose. While there is no indication that Victoria's Secret forced her to take the drug, these testimonies and revelations sent shockwaves through the Victoria's Secret fanbase, confirming as they did what many had long suspected: that the 'Angel body' wasn't always just the product of good genes and dedicated gym time, but instead could be borne out of extreme and, at times, unsafe practices.

The cracks in the glossy facade were becoming harder to ignore. Victoria's Secret began to feel increasingly out of touch, clinging to an outdated ideal while the rest of the industry embraced change, and there was a growing sense of discontent gaining traction online. The nail in Victoria's Secret's coffin came in late 2018, when former chief marketing officer Ed Razek told *Vogue* magazine that the brand had no interest in casting plus-size or transgender models in its fashion show. 'Shouldn't you have transsexuals in the show? No. No, I don't think we should,' he said, using an outdated term for transgender people. He cited the reason for the lack of plus-size models in the show being that the show was meant to be a 'fantasy'.

The idea of Victoria's Secret as a 'fantasy' is revealing. It begs the question: whose fantasy is it representative of, exactly? For decades, the brand sold women an image designed for the male gaze; an ideal shaped by Western beauty standards that prized youth, thinness and a kind of polished, performative sexiness. The women in the glossy campaigns were typically beautiful, confident and sensual. The so-called fantasy was never about women feeling powerful and comfortable in their own bodies; rather it was about being pleasing to look at.

The reaction to Razek's problematic remarks was strong and widespread, and the brand scrambled to redeem its reputation. Razek apologized and just months later Victoria's Secret hired its first transgender model, Valentina Sampaio, and cast its first ever curve model, Ali Tate Cutler. Despite these decisions signifying that the brand was attempting to take some small steps to being more inclusive, the moves ultimately felt performative and weren't enough to undo the damage caused: the same year, Razek resigned following public pressure, and the famous lingerie show was cancelled.

Following a six-year hiatus, the return of the Victoria's Secret show was announced in 2024. I had high hopes for what this new era of Victoria's Secret might bring, but the runway show was pretty lacklustre when it came to diversity: yes, it featured two trans models, Valentina Sampaio and Alex Consani, disproving Razek's remarks that there isn't a place for transgender models as a Victoria's Secret angel. But as I watched thin model after thin model appear on the runway, I realized that not much else had changed: what felt abundantly clear was that the brand didn't actually care much about inclusivity. There was a token attempt at showcasing body diversity with the inclusion of Ashley Graham and Paloma Elsesser, but both models are a very palatable take on 'plus size': more mid-size than plus, and both women embody the more conventionally attractive hourglass shape. What's more, both models were more covered up than their thinner counterparts: Paloma wore a dress, and Ashley wore a corset under a lacy robe. Their outfits seemed in contrast to the midriff-baring string two-pieces worn by the other, straight-size women. Paloma and Ashley aside, we were treated to a display of women who embody the same, very narrow lens of beauty that was so damaging to our formative minds: tall, tanned, extremely lean, with defined abs and zero cellulite. It felt just like the old days of Victoria's Secret.

Initially, I saw this as a missed opportunity for the brand to use its global stage to showcase a wide and varied range of beauty and body types and in turn make women across the world feel seen, celebrated and welcomed in a space from which they have always been excluded. There's no doubt that they did miss that opportunity, but in some ways, and as defeatist as it may sound, I wonder if it even matters anymore, given that, as a collective, our interest in body diversity has waned and we are once again craving thinness. Looking at the TikTok videos that surfaced following the show, showing girls eating ice to try and achieve the famous VS body type and reposting videos of the angels for 'motivation', it doesn't appear that the lack of diversity ended up being much of a bad thing for the brand.

Thin, But Not *Too* Thin

In 2023, Gwyneth Paltrow shared her now-infamous daily 'wellness routine' on the *The Art of Being Well* podcast: a daily regimen that included bone broth, IV drips, and sauna detoxes. Commenters on a TikTok video of the podcast were quick to question the limited number of calories that seemed to feature in Gwyneth's diet. It's true that what she outlined sounded extreme, and I believe we need to approach it with a healthy measure of critical thinking. The routine Gwyneth shared wouldn't be attainable for the vast majority of people in the world, and arguably, it wasn't healthy. What *was* interesting to see was the discomfort that Gwyneth's revelation stirred up – not just because it was (again, arguably) unhealthy, but because it was *revealing*. It pulled back the curtain on what it actually takes for women in Hollywood to maintain the body type that the industry demands of them – especially into their forties and fifties. Our society demands that this is done with ease and without effort, and Gwyneth had broken the unspoken contract: women are supposed to appear effortlessly thin.

Despite all this pressure, though, critics are quick to jump in with judgement when people are perceived as being *too* thin. First, Ariana Grande, and later her co-stars of *Wicked*, Cynthia Erivo and Michelle Yeoh, became the subject of relentless speculation during the *Wicked* press tours of 2025. After Grande appeared in paparazzi photos and interviews looking thinner after the release of the first film, social media erupted with concern – or perhaps more accurately, a barrage of judgement *disguised* as concern. Comments flooded in about her appearance: 'She looks so ill', 'She's way too thin', 'She's got an eating disorder'.

This example feels particularly insidious, because diagnosing a woman with an eating disorder based on photos or clips is not compassion, it's intrusion. Health is deeply personal and often invisible, and we simply do not know what someone is going through, what they're healing from, or how they're coping. Speculating about someone's health – especially in *such* a public way – doesn't help, but it can harm. It's invasive and cruel and not our business.

This pattern is nothing new, though. If Ariana represents the current version of this scrutiny, then Victoria Beckham is the longstanding poster girl. She has been a favourite target of our society's harsh judgement for decades. *Too thin, too obsessed with her appearance, too posh, too pouty, too serious . . .* Her body and face have been dissected for public consumption since her Spice Girls days when headlines called her 'Skeletal Spice' and questioned whether she was setting a bad example for girls.

She's been accused of starving herself, then mocked for being 'uptight' and never smiling. We've hungrily speculated on her calorie intake for decades as if knowing what Victoria Beckham eats for lunch is the secret to inner peace, and when her husband David revealed (perhaps inadvertently) on a podcast that 'Since I've met Victoria, she only eats grilled fish, steamed vegetables . . . She'll rarely deviate away from there. The only time that she's ever probably shared something that's been on my plate was actually when she was pregnant with Harper', the internet lost its mind.

The criticism levelled against her for this admission (that wasn't even hers!) was intense: she's setting a bad example, this is sad and unhealthy, nobody should live like this, she's everything that's wrong with celebrity culture . . . And we all forget that she was weighed live on TV just twelve weeks after giving birth, to check that her weight was 'back to normal'. In case you missed it, and hopefully you did, this happened on TV show *TFI Friday* in 1999. Wouldn't experiences like this, along with a level of media scrutiny we can probably never even fully imagine, have an effect on your body image and what you ate, too?

She isn't allowed to evolve, either: in a 2022 interview with *Grazia,* Victoria shared: 'It's an old-fashioned attitude, wanting to be really thin. I think women today want to be healthy, and curvy. They want to have some boobs, and a bum.' The criticism of this interview was scathing. People were livid that after years of epitomising the ultra-thin aesthetic, she was now seemingly endorsing curves. She was accused of hypocrisy and performative empowerment.

While I understand this reaction, I strongly believe that it is counterproductive to progress. A woman trying to speak from a new place – possibly a softer one, maybe a more self-aware one – should be met, in my opinion, with curiosity and compassion, not outrage. If not, how are any of us supposed to evolve?

The Politics of Thinness

This returned desire towards thinness in recent years has undoubtedly coincided with a wider political and cultural swing back toward more conservative values. There's an increased push for women to return to their 'traditional' roles with the rise of the 'trad wife', where women with vast audiences on social media romanticise a 1950s-style life of domesticity, baking bread in floral aprons, keeping an immaculate home and serving their husbands. On the surface, this is framed as a personal choice, even as a form of empowerment, standing for a rejection of the pressures of modern capitalism in favour of something 'simpler'. Scratching the surface, though, these influencers often reflect a worldview in which women's primary value lies in service: to their families, their husbands, their homes. Many of them also present motherhood as an integral part of the aesthetic, invariably maintaining impossibly slim bodies, despite their seemingly constant pregnancies and multiple children. The image of Hannah Neeleman – a former ballerina turned popular 'trad wife' influencer and mother of eight – competing in a beauty pageant less than two weeks after giving birth to her youngest child captures this paradox perfectly.

The 'trad wife' is a vision of femininity that's small, quiet, obedient and contained. Our bodies are not immune to or excluded from that ideology – in fact, the return of thinness fits neatly into it. What we're seeing isn't anything new: throughout history, every time women have gained ground, whether through increased rights or greater political sway, there's been a counter-pressure to shrink them, both literally and figuratively. As women gained the right to vote in 1920 and began pushing social boundaries – wearing shorter hemlines, smoking in public, and working outside the home – the body *du jour* became boyish and waif-like. Curves were out; a flat chest and narrow hips were now required. The same pattern re-emerged in the 1990s, in the wake of second-wave feminism and a growing female presence in boardrooms, politics and media, with fashion responding with the embracing of 'heroin chic' and an aesthetic of fragility.

The pursuit of thinness makes us both physically and mentally smaller: it consumes vast amounts of time, energy, money and mental space. Counting calories, tracking steps, obsessing over portion sizes, planning workouts, scrutinising our reflections: it's a full-time job that leaves little room for anything else. When women are preoccupied with shrinking their bodies, they have less capacity to expand into other areas of life – whether that's political activism, creative ambition or professional advancement. Thinness becomes not just a beauty standard but a form of social control; a way to keep women busy, compliant and constantly self-critical.

Now, we're back here again. Thin really is back in, and, if I'm honest, this period has been really difficult, both personally and professionally. My work revolves around body image, and over the past couple of years, social media has started to feel like a hostile place for those of us pushing back against the thin ideals. Where I was once overwhelmingly met with curiosity, celebration, and even relief from my audience, I now find myself encountering more scepticism, defensiveness and outright trolling than ever before. Posts that celebrate body diversity are inevitably met with comments about 'promoting obesity' and an 'unhealthy lifestyle', and nuanced conversations about weight and health are reduced to strawman arguments.

Don't get me wrong: there are lots of people still craving the kind of content I produce, who let me know that the work I do has helped them on their own personal journeys of unlearning years of body shame. Those messages mean everything to me, as does the fact that you are here, now, reading this book; still engaging in this kind of content even though it's no longer 'in fashion'. Despite what our social media feeds may be telling us, real people are still living in real bodies; still trying to learn to accept ourselves exactly as we are; still trying not to cave under the relentless pressure we seem to be facing from every angle to conform to stereotypes of thinness and prescribed beauty. That said, I'd be lying if I said I wasn't nervous to show up online these days, or even to be writing this book. Posting about body image makes me anxious because I know that, right now, it goes against the grain. The pendulum is firmly in the other direction and pushing against it is not only scary but exhausting – not just because of the backlash itself, but because it's a stark reminder of how quickly cultural tides can turn, and how fragile progress really is. I sometimes feel like we've been pushed back a decade overnight, and that all the work we did and progress we made has just vanished into thin air.

The stakes have also never been higher. As frivolous as beauty and body image may seem on the surface, we're not just talking about aesthetics or trends here; we're talking about health and, in some cases, lives. In the US, health visits for eating disorders among children under the age of seventeen more than doubled between 2018 and 2022.[5] In England, hospital admissions for mental health among girls aged 11–15 shot up by a staggering 113 per cent, and admissions related to eating disorders increased by 515 per cent during the same period.[6] Meanwhile, NHS data shows that the prevalence of eating disorders among 11–16-year-olds rose from 0.5 per cent in 2017 to 2.6 per cent in 2023, and among 17–19-year-olds, that figure rose from 0.8 per cent to 12.5 per cent.[7]

It's not just about self-esteem and health, though: thinness has long carried social and economic power. Studies have shown that thin women are often perceived as more competent, more disciplined and more employable than their peers, and these perceptions translate into real financial advantage. Research cited by *The Economist* found that 'overweight' women earn around 10 per cent less than thinner women, and that the wage premium for a master's degree (roughly 18 per cent) is only about twice as large as the income boost a woman could theoretically gain by losing around 65 lb. In other words, being thin can sometimes be almost as financially rewarding as further education. The gross unfairness of that gap is stark. Weight has no bearing on intelligence, creativity, leadership or work ethic, yet it continues to shape how women are perceived and valued in the workplace. These numbers show the strength of our collective bias: thinness is still read as a sign of discipline and self-control, while fatness is unfairly equated with laziness or lack of willpower.

Crucially, these costly assumptions are not applied equally. Studies show that men don't face the same financial penalty for being heavier – in some cases, the opposite is true. Research from the *Journal of Applied Psychology* found that bigger men were often perceived as more powerful and competent, while heavier women were penalized and paid less.[8] It's a shocking reminder of how differently we view the same body through the lens of gender: a man's size may be perceived as signs of strength, authority, and leadership, whereas a woman's size is all-too-often connected to weakness or lack of control. The very traits celebrated in men are punished in women.

Nowhere is this double standard more obvious – or more absurd, frankly – than in how we respond to 'mixed-weight relationships': relationships where there is a noticeable size difference between partners. For those in the public eye, the scrutiny is fierce. When a bigger woman dates a man, commentary explodes: *He's a hero! Does he have a fetish?* The woman is forced to justify the relationship's legitimacy; she can't simply be in love, she must explain how she managed to 'snare' her man. Meanwhile, a heavier man with a thin partner is treated as normal, or even endearing, and not worthy of a headline or a moral panic.

We see this over and over again: Seth Rogen, Jonah Hill, Vince Vaughn, Jack Black – men who are in bigger bodies (and yes, some only slightly so) often paired, both on-screen and off, with thin love interests, and *no one bats an eyelid*. The underlying message is clear: men can be loved for their humour, charm, talent or status. Women, however? They must earn love through physical perfection.

The same is true in fictional settings too. Think of *The King of Queens, According to Jim, Family Guy, Modern Family* and *The Simpsons*. In each of these, the dynamic is the same: a heavier, often goofy or underachieving man is paired with a slim, conventionally attractive woman. And we never question it! He gets to be funny, flawed and lovable. She gets to be thin.

The cruellest part is that we internalize this; we start to question ourselves in our own relationships. 'Do we look right together?' 'Do people think he could do better?' We see love, or even affection, as something we have to *deserve* through our bodies. It speaks to the larger issue of the emotional labour women do just to exist in the world – monitoring not just their own feelings, but the perceptions of everyone around them.

It's vital that we share and discuss the realities of the world we're living in now. The statistics and the data paint a very sobering picture of where we are and why all of this is so important. These body 'trends' are doing so much harm, and they're the very reason why I can't – and won't – stop. If anything, the pushback I receive for my work makes me even more determined to keep showing up; to keep creating space for these very important conversations; to keep reminding people that their worth has nothing at all to do with the size of their bodies.

The Headlines
- We saw some progress as a result of the mainstream body positivity movement, but much of this was rapidly reversed once thinness became profitable for corporations again, turning our bodies into a fashion trend
- The return of thinness isn't a coincidence; it sits within a broader cultural swing towards conservative values, traditional gender roles and a shrinking vision of womanhood
- The stakes are real: rates of eating disorders are rising sharply, especially amongst girls and teenagers, and thinness continues to grant women measurable social and economic advantages

A Moment of Reflection
- *When did I first learn that 'thin' meant 'good'? Who taught me that?*
- *How often do I conflate 'health' with 'morality'?*
- *In what ways have I internalized or participated in the return of thinness, even subtly?*
- *What media or accounts actually make me feel neutral or good about my body? Which ones quietly prompt comparison and negative feelings?*
- *If I weren't trying to take up less space, physically or metaphorically, what could I do with that reclaimed energy?*

Where Do We Go From Here?

Culture is cyclical, but having an awareness of this fact breaks the loop for us as individuals. Every time we name what's happening, and refuse to buy back into it, we weaken the forces profiting from our self-doubt. The thin ideal may have resurfaced, but this time, we see it for what it is – and that is powerful. It enables us to fight back and to see that the problem is not with us and our bodies, but rather, with the systems that promote these ideals.

Chapter 2

The Ozempic Effect

Hollywood's worst-kept secret used to be plastic surgery, then along came Ozempic. Originally formulated as a treatment for type-2 diabetes, in mid-2021 the drug was approved by the FDA for weight loss, and soon it had slipped into celebrity 'wellness' routines and, one ultra-thin red carpet at a time, it quietly began to redefine the beauty ideal, until suddenly, it wasn't so quiet anymore. A secret too groundbreaking to gatekeep, the drug quickly spilled out of celebrity circles and into the mainstream: it was widely rumoured that Kim Kardashian had used Ozempic to shed 16 lb in three weeks to fit into Marilyn Monroe's iconic and objectively *tiny* dress for the 2022 Met Gala – a rumour she has neither confirmed nor denied – while Elon Musk revealed the 'secret' to his 'fit, ripped and healthy' new look was 'fasting and Wegovy'. The injection subsequently stormed TikTok, emerging as a trend on the platform that had amassed over 300 million views by November 2022. Social media platforms exploded with personal stories, before and after photos, as well as hacks to source the drug.

Meanwhile, the media rushed to hail GLP-1s as a revolutionary weapon in the 'battle against the bulge', with the drugs being lauded as one of the most effective additions *ever* in the ongoing 'fight against obesity'. All this inevitably led to a huge increase in public interest – along with a worldwide shortage of semaglutide, prompting serious concerns for diabetic patients who rely on the medication for its original use. By the end of that year, Ozempic was the word on *everyone's* lips.

Dieting Culture and Food Noise

For decades, we've been sold the idea that weight loss is a matter of willpower: calories in, calories out; self-control is king. That's not just a belief that's shaped diet culture and general cultural beliefs either; it's also deeply embedded in medical systems too. People in larger bodies have long reported being dismissed by doctors, with symptoms attributed automatically to their weight. Coming to a doctor with a knee injury? It must be your weight! Fatigued? Try a diet. This kind of weight stigma leads to missed diagnoses, delayed treatment and poorer outcomes overall. If you found yourself unable to lose weight through diet and exercise, or if you couldn't maintain weight loss, the implication was clear and, actually, fairly explicit: you'd failed. You lacked discipline, you just weren't trying hard enough. But that narrative has *always* been flawed. 'For a long time, we've treated obesity as a moral failing rather than a complex biological condition,' explains Dr Giles Yeo, geneticist and obesity researcher at the University of Cambridge. 'The truth is, body weight is determined by a host of factors – genetics, environment, psychology – and not everyone has the same biological starting point.'

For many people, weight is not just about willpower. It's biological, psychological, environmental and hormonal. The body actively resists weight loss, adjusting its metabolism and ramping up hunger hormones in ways that make sustained change incredibly difficult. 'When you lose weight, your brain isn't happy – it hates it,' Giles explains. 'No matter what size you are, when you lose weight, your brain recognizes that you're losing fuel stores, and it fights back. It increases your hunger, lowers your metabolism so you burn fewer calories, and it becomes harder and harder to keep the weight off. Anyone who's dieted will know that the moment you start dieting, you feel hungry. That's your brain trying to stop you from losing weight and dragging you back to where you were before. That's just how the body is wired.'

It's not just the physical resistance that makes weight loss difficult: it's also the mental toll. Many people, including myself, live with something called 'food noise': a constant, internal chatter about eating and a preoccupation with food. I am intimately familiar with the idea of food noise. For as long as I can remember, it has played in the background of my brain – at times, a low-level hum, and at others, a deafening roar. It sounds something like this: *'I can't believe it's so long until dinner, I'm already hungry . . . Or am I? Wait, think about it, Al – are you actually hungry or is this emotional hunger? Should I have a snack? I really want a cookie. Do I really, though? Yes, I do. But that's not exactly a nutritious snack, is it? I want it really badly, though. OK, I'm going to have one. Now I want another one . . . Do I? But what if I want one after dinner instead? And: surely I can't have three cookies in a day? Maybe I should just have a yoghurt. OK, now I'm full and satisfied! Oh wow, look at that sandwich in the deli window, I really want that! Maybe I am still hungry. Maybe I need something savoury instead? But dinner is only two hours away, should I just wait? No, I don't think I can wait, I'm hungry. But am I?'*

It may sound intense, but that's because it is. Food noise is draining; it's consuming, and it's often relentless. And honestly, it's hard to admit all of this, because it feels like I'm confessing to something deeply shameful. Women, in particular, are taught that thinking about food too much is unseemly; that appetite is something to suppress or hide. To say that food occupies this much mental space feels embarrassing. But I know it's important to share because, if I experience it, the chances are many of you reading this book do too.

I asked Dr Giles for his expert definition of food noise: 'Food noise is thinking about food constantly – even when you're not hungry. I have it – when I am full straight after lunch, I am already planning dinner in my head.' I also questioned Giles about the link between food noise and dieting, because I have always believed, in my admittedly non-expert opinion, that food noise is a result of dieting. While he was careful not to oversimplify a complicated phenomenon, he agreed that dieting does at the very least exacerbate food noise. 'Being hungry makes you think about food,' he explained. 'And dieting makes you feel hungry. So yes, it increases food noise. It's probably too simplistic to say that dieting *causes* food noise, but it undeniably turns the volume up.'

Jane Ogden, a Professor of Health Psychology, makes a similar point. She explains that 'chronic dieting involves setting boundaries around food and trying to eat less. This often creates a rebound effect and a sense of preoccupation with the very foods trying to be denied. It therefore makes food noise worse as we think about it even more.'

But the noise doesn't come from hunger alone: it's fuelled by the constant, contradictory messages we receive about food and bodies. We're told to eat 'clean' but not to be obsessive; to enjoy food, but not too much; to 'treat ourselves', but compensate for it with exercise or later deprivation. What's more, the language we use around food – calling dessert a 'guilty pleasure' or describing something rich as 'naughty' or 'indulgent' – illustrates how moralised eating has become. As Jane puts it, 'food has become very contaminated with black and white thinking and is classified into good vs bad, healthy vs unhealthy, treat vs necessary, and therefore often comes with a sense of shame or judgement. This heightens the amount we think about food and can cause food noise as food becomes laden with emotions which are often negative.'

We absorb the idea that some foods are 'good' and others are 'bad' and that our worth fluctuates depending on what's on our plate. Is it any wonder so many of us are caught in a loop of craving, shame and restriction?

The acknowledgement that food noise is a side effect of diet culture makes clear that it's not our fault for experiencing it; we've been conditioned to think about food constantly through chronic dieting that rewires our relationship with hunger, fullness and trust in our bodies. All that makes weight loss even more difficult, when our minds and bodies are rebelling against the process on a physiological level – and that's where GLP-1s have changed the game.

The Impact of GLP-1s

Now feels like a good time to explore the drug itself: what *is* a GLP-1, how does it work, and why has it become one of the most talked-about, in-demand drugs to hit the pharmaceutical industry in decades? One of the most popular and well-known of these, Ozempic, was originally developed to treat type-2 diabetes. It works by mimicking a naturally occurring hormone in the gut called GLP-1 (Glucagon-Like Peptide-1) that plays a key role in regulating appetite and blood sugar. 'Semaglutide makes you feel fuller faster and for longer through both mimicking GLP-1 and delaying gastric emptying, i.e. slowing digestion,' explains Giles. 'All of this means that you don't feel as hungry, so it turns down the volume on food noise.'

Essentially, it takes away the constant internal battle of food noise and stops users from obsessing over their next meal. 'The reduction of food noise was the biggest driver for me in taking Mounjaro,' influencer Sasha Pallari told me. She deliberated long and hard about taking a GLP-1 – 'I don't even like taking paracetamol for a headache!' – but the allure of quieting the constant, obsessive chatter around food was deeply compelling. 'To have help with a problem that has consumed my thoughts for most of my life felt like a kind of miracle cure,' she said. When she did start, the effect was immediate. 'It worked instantly. It felt like someone had taken a weight off my shoulders and cleared the path in front of me. Eight months on, I estimate that my food noise has overall reduced by about 70 per cent.' This cognitive relief from an obsession with food is what has been life-changing for so many people who have taken some form of GLP-1. Having lived with the exhausting background hum of food noise for so long, no longer needing ironclad self-control to fight against it is revolutionary. But here's the thing: who actually gets to experience that relief?

There's a huge financial privilege involved with taking weight-loss drugs, and for those who can't afford the costs, many are turning to a booming black market that provides pens from dodgy websites, splitting doses with friends, or swapping tips on Telegram groups on how to fake a qualifying diagnosis. When supply runs low, desperate patients mix leftover doses themselves or ration injections to stretch them out. While all this is happening behind closed doors, the companies behind these drugs are posting record-breaking profits. Novo Nordisk, the maker of Ozempic and Wegovy, became Europe's most valuable company in 2023, overtaking luxury empires like LVMH and becoming more profitable than entire national economies.

Analysts call it 'the Ozempic effect'. Rival companies like Eli Lilly, which makes GLP-1 injections Mounjaro and Zepbound, are racing to keep up, pouring billions into new manufacturing plants and marketing campaigns to meet demand – because if we know one thing for sure, it's that weight loss sells. We're desperate, and the commercial forces at play know it. Yes, they're selling medication, but on a wider level they're selling hope, control, and, ultimately, a higher value in society. That 'higher value' is a tangible and measurable advantage. Studies consistently show that thinner people are treated better, earn more and receive better medical care. As we explored in Chapter 1, one study found that women classified as 'obese' earn, on average, 10 per cent less than thinner women doing the same job.[9] All this means that what these drugs promise runs deeper than just weight loss and thinner bodies; it promises a social advantage and an escape from the stigma and judgement that fatphobia still carries.

These companies are tapping into a collective anxiety that's been carefully and consistently nurtured for decades: the fear of taking up too much space, of not fitting in or conforming to the beauty standards we're sold.

And all this means that we're willing to pay – and we pay a lot. These injections don't come cheap: in the UK, private prescriptions for weight-loss injections typically cost between £150 and £300 per month and, for many, these drugs are needed indefinitely to maintain the weight loss (we'll get onto that . . .) and keep the food noise at bay. Some people qualify for prescriptions via the NHS, but many don't meet the strict criteria and waiting lists are long. Even for those who do, there are waiting lists, supply shortages and endless hoops to jump through to keep the prescriptions coming. In the US, prices are significantly higher, with costs ranging from $900 to $1300 per month depending on insurance coverage. And even insurance coverage isn't a guarantee! Many US insurers only cover these drugs for a limited time – sometimes as little as six months – before cutting patients off, leaving them to either pay out of pocket or stop treatment altogether.

To make things even more precarious, prices are changing rapidly. In September 2025, manufacturer Eli Lilly increased the list price for a month's supply of the highest dose of Mounjaro from £122 to £330.

But here's the thing: these drugs won't cost this much forever. Currently, Novo Nordisk holds exclusive rights to make and sell semaglutide. That monopoly ends when the primary patent expires, which is currently expected to be in around 2032. 'When Ozempic goes off patent, its price could drop to around £10 a month,' explains Giles. 'Other pharmaceutical companies will be able to legally manufacture and sell generic versions, and generic versions are usually significantly cheaper than brand-name versions – sometimes by 70–90 per cent less.'

I wonder how that shift might impact us. If these drugs become cheap and widely available, how widespread will the usage become, and just how normalized will it become to silence our hunger? What will that do to the way we think about food, our bodies and our health, and what happens to the people who choose not to take them – or who can't take them? Will not taking a drug to lose weight start to feel like a rebellion in and of itself? It's hard to say, but what is already clear is just how effective these drugs can be. For many, the silencing of food noise has led to dramatic weight loss without the relentless effort of dieting. In clinical trials, people lost an average of 15 per cent[10] of their body weight with semaglutide, and up to 22 per cent[11] with newer drugs like tirzepatide, found in Mounjaro or Zepbound. This is far more than what's typically seen with 'lifestyle changes' alone, but of course, it's not that simple.

The rise of these drugs has also brought with it a growing list of potential side effects. Nausea, vomiting, diarrhoea, and constipation are common, but in some cases, they can be severe. Some users have developed gastroparesis, or stomach paralysis, a condition where the stomach stops emptying properly, leading to chronic pain and vomiting. Lawsuits have already been filed with patients claiming long-term gastrointestinal damage, and there are other physical concerns, too: links to pancreatitis, kidney issues, and even certain types of cancer, although the research is still developing and evolving as more data emerges. 'While GLP-1s appear to be largely safe, as with any drug, there are side effects,' says Giles. 'These drugs are powerful, and while they work incredibly well for some, they're not without risks, especially if used long-term or outside of a clinical setting.' Giles argues, however, that for some people the risk of taking weight-loss drugs must be weighed up against the risk of *not* taking it. 'There might be evidence that it increases the risk of certain cancers, but it can also potentially decrease the risk of a lot of cancer by reducing weight, insulin sensitivity and inflammation, all of which can be factors associated with cancer risk.'

In other words, the conversation around GLP-1s isn't black and white – it's nuanced, medical, and deeply individual. In the public eye, though, inevitably, that nuance is often lost. While experts weigh long-term risks and benefits, much of the mainstream conversation has been shaped by celebrity influence rather than clinical guidance. Now, some of those same celebrities who helped catapult drugs like Ozempic into public consciousness are beginning to share their own cautionary tales. During a June 2023 chat with Andy Cohen, Amy Schumer revealed she had tried Ozempic 'about a year ago' but stopped shortly after due to its side effects. 'I was one of those people who felt sick – I couldn't even play with my son,' she said. Despite noticing some weight loss, Amy said the side effects made it not worth continuing the drug.

Actor Stephen Fry shared that he tried Ozempic on his doctor's recommendation, but it didn't go as planned. 'In the first week, I thought, "This is amazing. I don't want to eat or drink any alcohol. This is going to be fantastic",' he recalled in March 2024. 'But then I started to feel ill, and it just got worse. I was throwing up four or five times a day, and I realized, "I can't do this". So that was the end of it.'

Model Lottie Moss, meanwhile, spoke on a podcast about how she was rushed to hospital and suffered a seizure after she took excessively high doses of Ozempic, which she admitted to acquiring 'below board'. 'This is a warning to everyone,' she said. 'Please, if you're thinking of taking it, do not take it, it's so not worth it.'

Outside of the spotlight, the stories are often even more sobering. A growing number of lawsuits have been filed in the US against two pharmaceutical companies that produce weight-loss injections: Novo Nordisk and Eli Lilly. They allege that the drugs can trigger non-arteritic anterior ischaemic optic neuropathy, a condition that occurs when blood flow to the optic nerve is blocked or reduced, and can lead to blindness. There are also ongoing cases against both companies alleging that the drugs had caused instances of gastroparesis, or stomach paralysis, which impacts digestion. The companies have refuted the claims.

Someone close to me, who has asked to remain anonymous, tried Mounjaro, hoping for relief from the constant mental battle with food and weight management – just like Sasha Pallari experienced. Instead, they came away calling it (in their own words) 'poison'.

'I thought it would make life easier,' she told me. 'Instead, I felt like I was living in the bathroom. I had diarrhoea every few hours – sometimes all through the night – and these horrible sulphur burps that made me gag. Food made me sick, but not eating also made me sick . . . I was so miserable.' She added: 'The nausea was constant. The vomiting was so bad I couldn't even keep water down some days. It felt like I was injecting myself with poison, but I continued for four weeks at the lowest dose, until it reached a point where I wasn't able to leave the house, and I knew I had to stop. I felt a huge sense of relief when it was finally all out of my system.'

Such is the allure of weight loss, however, that she actually decided to try the drug again a few weeks later, once she was feeling better. 'I know that's quite shocking, and everyone around me tried to stop me, but when my appetite returned, it returned with a vengeance, and I panicked that I'd put on what I'd lost so I gave it another go. I was desperate both to not gain the weight I'd lost but also to lose more weight, and this felt like my only option.' Unfortunately, her experience the second time around wasn't any better: in fact, it resulted in a public mishap when she couldn't get to a toilet in time. I won't say any more.

Physical symptoms aside, there is also the psychological impact of using weight-loss injections: many patients report developing disordered eating patterns, anxiety around food, and an overwhelming fear of regaining weight once they stop taking the drugs – all side effects of this 'miracle cure' that are rarely discussed or acknowledged. For some, GLP-1s have been life-changing, but for others, these drugs have replaced one kind of struggle with another. And that's the part that doesn't fit neatly into the headlines or the before-and-after photos: the fact that, for all the hype, GLP-1s haven't necessarily freed us from the burden of managing our weight, they've just changed the rules of the game.

After Weight-loss Drugs . . .

One of the more difficult truths about GLP-1 drugs that we haven't touched on yet is the sobering fact that, for many, they don't offer a true 'cure' from weight gain. As a result, many users may need to stay on the drugs indefinitely to maintain the weight they've lost, because once the drug stops, so does the weight loss – and very often, the lost weight returns. One study determined that stopping GLP-1s leads to a return to a starting weight in less than two years, and the rate of regain is greater than observed following behavioural weight-management programmes – that is, diets, essentially.[12]

'These drugs are very effective at helping you lose weight, but when you stop them, weight regain is much faster than [after stopping] diets,' said researcher Professor Susan Jebb. 'Either people really have to accept this as a treatment for life, you're going to have to keep going forever, or we in science need to think really, really hard, how to support people when they stop the drug.'

The current NICE (National Institute for Health and Care Excellence) guidelines recommend that patients in the UK use weight-loss drugs for a maximum of two years. But the science, and the experience of real people, tells us that stopping after that period is rarely simple. For many, it isn't just weight that rebounds, but hunger and food noise and a fear of weight regain.

Giles explains why: 'GLP-1s are a drug, and like all drugs, they only work when you're taking them. Your hormone levels return to normal and your body is reset to where you were, and your brain begins to try dragging your weight back up – just like it does on a diet. Hunger returns, food noise creeps back in and the body fights to return to its previous set point.' I asked Giles whether taking a GLP-1 means committing for life. 'I think that the majority of people who are taking the drugs will need to be on some version of them for a long time,' he says.

The reality is something I've seen play out. A close friend of mine, who asked to remain anonymous, came off Mounjaro after several months of use. At first, she said, she felt fine, and was hopeful about ending her experience with the drug. 'My appetite was still small for a while, and I told myself I'd just "eat mindfully" and keep the weight off,' she told me. But she soon noticed subtle changes: her hunger started to return, with portion sizes becoming bigger and the number of snacks between meals increasing.

Then, when the drug had completely left her system, everything hit at once. 'I felt *totally* out of control around food,' she said. 'It was like the food noise came back louder than ever – I'd wake up thinking about breakfast, then immediately start worrying about what I'd eat next. I felt possessed by food again, but the preoccupation felt even more intense than it had been before I started taking Mounjaro.'

She described a sense of rising panic about weight regain. 'I was quickly regaining the weight and I felt so sad because so many people had commented on my weight loss and said how much better I was looking,' she said. She was, ultimately, scared of losing that validation, that feeling of being seen differently. She'd also bought a new wardrobe to accommodate her smaller size, and it was quickly becoming redundant. 'I felt like I was failing.'

My friend had been buying the drug from an online pharmacy rather than a medical expert, so there was no professional support available for her in this time. She ended up starting to take the drug again, and I'll be honest: I don't blame her. It sounds like an impossible situation to be in – feeling like your body is rebelling while you panic, and no guidance from the system that made the drug so easy to access in the first place. I can see how people end up reverting back to taking it again.

Some users don't plan to stop at all, which is the case for Sasha Pallari: 'I have no intention to stop – and so long as my doctors and other medical professionals say it's OK, I will keep taking them. I feel that, in itself, speaks volumes to how much they've changed and helped me in life.'

This doesn't definitively mean there's no room for change using GLP-1s, though. 'I do think there's an opportunity for some people to use the drug as a sort of reset,' says Giles. 'When the food noise quiets and the physiological drive to eat is dialled down, it can create space to build new habits, new patterns and perhaps a better relationship with food. And for some, that foundation may help them maintain progress even after coming off the drug.' Still, he cautions that this isn't the norm and that framing GLP-1s as temporary or willpower-boosting tools overlooks the reality of how weight biology works for most people.

In the Spotlight

When a trend originates within the top of the social hierarchy – the rich and famous – it rarely stays there. Weight-loss drugs are a perfect illustration of this: what began as a private prescription within celebrity circles trickled down through the layers of culture until it became a mainstream aspiration.

The Price of Pretty

When Jimmy Kimmel opened the 2023 Oscars ceremony, he looked out at the A-list crowd and asked: 'I can't help but wonder, "Is Ozempic right for me?".' The crowd went . . . mild. The joke was perhaps a bit too close to home, judging by the noticeably thinner silhouettes of that year's attendees. I can't help but suspect that the audience's lacklustre reaction might have been indicative of something that no one was quite ready to admit: that this time, the transformation wasn't just down to Pilates, juice cleanses and plenty of water.

Despite the already-thin Hollywood circle becoming noticeably thinner, celebrities weren't exactly forthcoming about admitting to using the drug. This is both unsurprising and understandable, given the pressure – on women in particular – to be thin and stay thin without appearing to make any effort, as well as the shame that accompanies any weight-loss methods that are viewed as a 'quick fix' or the 'easy way out', as GLP-1s are. There's a strange, cultural hierarchy of weight loss: suffering somehow earns you more credit. Sweating it out at the gym, resisting dessert, counting every single calorie: these are all seen as signs of discipline, self-control and even virtue and something worth celebrating and rewarding. But taking a weekly injection? That's seen as cheating. It skips the struggle – and in our culture, struggle is seen as proof of a woman's worth.

This belief that our bodies must be worked for; that thinness must be earned, reinforces stigma around GLP-1 use, but it also exposes the wider expectation that women should meet beauty standards through struggle. Effort makes thinness more admirable – but, of course, that effort must be quiet and graceful and without complaint. It's impossible.

Meanwhile, men move through these conversations with far more ease. Elon Musk casually tweeted about using Wegovy and was treated like he'd discovered a cool hack. Leonardo DiCaprio can fluctuate in size and still be hailed as a sex symbol with a cute 'dad bod'. No one's writing op-eds about whether he's 'let himself go'. Men's bodies are rarely politicised, never moralised and almost always forgiven.

With all this in mind, I must be honest and admit that, if I was a celebrity, I probably wouldn't confess to using it publicly either – the risk for a woman is too high. Still, a few voices started to speak up. American actress Kathy Bates shared that, having lost around 80 lb through significant diet and lifestyle changes, she'd lost an additional 20 lb using Ozempic. A fair few reality TV stars of the *Real Housewives* franchises admitted to taking weight-loss drugs. *Real Housewives of New Jersey* star Dolores Catania confirmed she was taking Mounjaro to lose weight at the series' end of season show, telling Andy Cohen during an appearance on *Watch What Happens Live* that 'I wasn't going to come to the reunion looking any bigger than anyone else, so I got on the bandwagon.' There's a lot to unpack there, and it's a tough quote to reflect on. Given the context of her work, though, I absolutely understand this mentality, and the notion of suddenly finding yourself bigger than everyone else because of weight-loss injections is a subject I'll come back to.

Perhaps the biggest star to talk about their experience of taking GLP-1s is Oprah Winfrey. It was a controversial thing for Oprah to reveal, given her very public relationship with dieting and her own body image, and I have complicated feelings around it, as do many others, no doubt, so let's explore. Oprah has been incredibly open about her weight fluctuations during her decades-long career: you may well have heard of the infamous 1988 stunt that involved her dragging a wagon full of animal fat across the stage to represent how much weight she'd lost (67 lb) on a liquid-only diet. The unsettling moment, watched by a staggering 62 million viewers, which translated to one in four Americans, became a defining and controversial pop culture landmark, and a stark reflection of our society's almost pathological obsession with weight. Oprah has since admitted that the stunt was one of the biggest regrets of her career, a powerful confession that hinted at a shifting perspective. Despite that, though, she remained closely tied to the weight-loss industry. In 2015, Oprah partnered with Weight Watchers (now WW), joining the company's board of directors and acquiring a 10 per cent stake in the company.

In what felt like a sharp pivot from years of promoting willpower-based weight loss, Oprah told *People* magazine in 2023 that she had been taking weight-loss medication, having realized that weight management isn't simply a matter of self-control. 'The fact that there's a medically approved prescription for managing weight and staying healthier, in my lifetime, feels like relief, like redemption, like a gift, and not something to hide behind and once again be ridiculed for,' she said. 'I'm absolutely done with the shaming from other people and particularly myself. I now use it as I feel I need it, as a tool to manage not yo-yo-ing.'

Whew. First off, I think Oprah's transparency here deserves credit. It's brave and vulnerable, especially given she was, at this point, still tied to a company whose core philosophy centred on self-discipline and restraint. This admission also sparked backlash, though – much of which I agree with. For nearly a decade, Oprah was the face of Weight Watchers (now WW), a programme built on the premise that with enough willpower, anyone could lose weight and keep it off. She promoted it passionately to millions of people, many of them vulnerable and often desperate. She also profited enormously from that role, earning an estimated $221 million through the partnership.[13] In a 2016 commercial for the company, Oprah told the camera: 'At Weight Watchers, I don't have to choose between weight loss and living well. I live well while losing weight. It is easier than it's ever been, and not one day have I felt deprived.' She added: 'And most important: it WORKS.'

Now look, I don't mean to vilify Oprah here. Of course she's allowed to change her mind. She's human, and she's certainly not the only celebrity to have profited from the weight-loss industry. But I think her example is representative of a much wider cultural tension at play with traditional diet programmes and the rise of pharmaceutical solutions like Ozempic and other GLP-1s. It raises, I believe, important questions about responsibility, messaging, and the evolving narrative around weight and health – questions that the traditional weight-loss industry has scrambled to answer. Weight Watchers (now WW) has since launched its own prescription medication programme, integrating GLP-1 drugs into its offerings. Similarly, Noom, the app that once focused solely on cognitive behavioural weight loss, has also introduced a telehealth service providing access to weight-loss medications. These pivots go to show just how disruptive these drugs have been, forcing huge, long-standing players of the industry to either evolve or risk irrelevance in a market increasingly dominated by pharmaceuticals. Even with these strategic shifts, the impact is clear: in May 2025, Weight Watchers (now WW) filed for Chapter 11 bankruptcy protection in the US as part of a major financial restructure aimed to eliminate approximately $1.15 billion of debt – yet another striking reflection of how profoundly the rise of weight-loss medications has upended the traditional diet industry.

As the companies evolve, the faces of this new era of weight loss do, too. The diet industry has always relied on celebrity endorsement to sell transformation, and that same formula has extended into the Ozempic era. In August 2025, tennis champion Serena Williams was announced as the new face of Ro, a telehealth company offering access to GLP-1 weight-loss drugs. In the glossy adverts for the campaign, Serena was pictured injecting her body in various places; she talked at length in the accompanying interview about 'taking control' of her health and losing weight herself while using a GLP-1.

Her partnership with Ro drew swift criticism: many pointed out that her husband, Alexis Ohanian, sits on Ro's board of directors, raising uncomfortable questions about financial interest and conflict. Others were unsettled by what this new partnership represented: one of the most celebrated athletes in history – a woman whose body has long embodied power and strength and athletic excellence – was now fronting a product designed to make people smaller.

I was one of the people who criticized the campaign, not because I think Serena shouldn't have the right to make her own choices with her body – she absolutely should – but because of the impact of this campaign. When someone with her platform and influence promotes a product for weight loss, it is a public endorsement of a pharmaceutical drug. We're not talking about a probiotic or a fitness app; it's a prescription medication with very real side effects designed to alter the way your body regulates hunger and weight.

When a celebrity like Serena promotes it, the drug inevitably stops being seen as medical – something that should be guided by doctors and evidence – and starts being seen as aspirational – another consumer trend. It blurs the line between healthcare and marketing and the messaging shifts from 'this is a serious medication with risks and side effects' to 'this is what health and success looks like'. I don't think anyone could deny that that's dangerous.

What troubles me most is the message it sends: that even the most extraordinary of bodies – one that has defied limits, broken records, carried a baby and been a symbol of strength and possibility for women everywhere – still isn't enough unless it's smaller.

In the very advert promoting the drug, Serena said: 'I am a very good use case of how you can do everything – eat healthy, work out to the point of playing professional sport and getting to the finals of Wimbledon and the US Open – and still not be able to lose weight.' I thought this was such an interesting quote because to me, that doesn't reflect failure as she's implying here, it reflects biology. If even one of the greatest athletes in the world can't lose weight, maybe it's because she isn't supposed to? Maybe it's not her body that's the problem, rather our culture's impossible expectation that every body should shrink.

Serena isn't the only elite athlete to step into this glossy new weight-loss economy: Simone Biles, the most decorated American gymnast in history, one of the most decorated gymnasts of all time, became the face of pharmaceutical company Eli Lilly's global campaign for Mounjaro in 2025 alongside her mother, Nellie. It was framed as a campaign for people with type-2 diabetes, yet on the brand's website, they clarify: 'Simone Biles does not have type-2 diabetes. Simone and Nellie Biles do not take Mounjaro.'

The Currency of 'Thinness' and Fear of Being Left Behind

Evidently, it's not as clear-cut as the headlines would have us believe when it comes to weight-loss drugs, because while they *have* disrupted the decades-old idea that weight loss is simply a matter of personal responsibility, it's also revealed a more complicated truth that goes against the glossy headlines: there is no magic solution, no silver bullet. For many, these drugs have also triggered a new kind of fear: *what if everyone else gets smaller and I don't? What if I'm the last one left who's not in a thin body?*

This sums up the sentiment I'm hearing from my audience: multiple people in their friendship groups are taking GLP-1s, and they're worried about being 'left behind'. It creates a sense of feeling that perhaps they should take it too, despite not actually wanting to take the drug.

Here's the thing: thinness has always been a social currency, especially for women. Weight-loss drugs didn't invent that. But now, thinness is not just reserved for a select few with certain genetics or an abundance of discipline; it's becoming something closer to an expectation. That's what feels different in this era of Ozempic: thinness is not just admired, it's starting to feel compulsory, and there appears to be growing judgement around not taking it. If there's a quick and easy way to shrink, why wouldn't you? Why would you choose *not* to be thin? Pair that with the high street adverts for weight-loss jabs, the Instagram and TikTok videos of people showing off their GLP-1 transformations and the casual way in which it might get mentioned in the group chat, and the pressure feels relentless. It's a new kind of policing of bodies: it's buried in the language of health, self-care and modern medicine, but underneath it's the same old toxic message: *you'd be better if you were smaller.*

Again, the influence this is inevitably having on young people is so concerning. Teenagers are coming of age in a digital landscape that is saturated with filters, AI and the relentless messaging of 'SkinnyTok'. Now, they're also being exposed to weight-loss injections marketed with before-and-after 'glow-ups', and light-hearted videos about injecting your way to a 'better body'. If GLP-1s had been around when I was a teenager, I would have gone to any lengths to get my hands on them, and let's be frank: given how easy it can be to obtain a prescription today, I don't think it would have been that difficult. There are qualifying criteria, of course. The official line is that you need a BMI of at least 30 – which is the number on the scale at which 'overweight' switches to 'obese' in the UK – or a BMI of 27 for those with a weight-related medical condition who have tried to lose weight through diet and exercise. This is all in theory, but in practise, it's often far more flexible.

Online consultations take minutes, and some clinics ask for little more than self-reported height and weight. With booming demand and high profit margins, it's no surprise that some providers are willing to blur the boundaries of eligibility to keep up with the market; to turn a blind eye to collateral damage, so to speak. This is one of the most troubling aspects of the weight-loss drug phenomenon. When the bar for access is so low, it's not just going to people who have a genuine medical need for it, it also reaches those for whom it could be really harmful. I'm talking specifically here about vulnerable people, especially anyone with an active or previous eating disorder. It's already happening. I've talked to people over Instagram who have admitted to lying about their weight, and about their history with eating disorders, just to get hold of these drugs. It's a perfect storm: the pressure is loud; the system is easy to manipulate; and the praise for thinness is relentless. When society rewards weight loss at any cost and access to powerful medication comes with little scrutiny, it creates a deeply dangerous environment – especially for those already vulnerable.

I want to speak to readers directly here and be clear on two things: first, if you *are* taking a GLP-1 drug, that's absolutely OK, and I completely respect your decision. Your body is your body, and what you do with it is nobody's business but your own. Secondly, if you're not taking a GLP-1 but you're feeling the intense pressure to do so, please remember that this pressure is the result of society's toxic relationship with weight and thinness, and has nothing to do with you, your worth or your value. The healthiest thing you can do is to try to block out the noise and come back to what's truly right for *you*, *your* life and *your* body. Of course, this conversation gets more complex when medical advice from a professional is involved, and I'm not a doctor, so I can't tell you what to do. But I do want to remind you of this: you are allowed to ask questions. You are allowed to take time and demand more information and to make decisions that feel safe and right for you, not just for the sake of fitting in and looking a certain way.

I recognize that GLP-1s have been life-changing for people with diabetes to help manage blood sugar, and for people living in larger bodies to lower risk of heart disease and improve quality of daily life in meaningful ways. That matters and it can't be left out of this conversation. At the same time, though, I believe we *have* to question why these medications are being embraced so widely and so quickly, and what that says about our culture. We may pretend that it's solely about health, but I truly believe that we use 'health' as a kind of moral disguise for our culture's obsession with thinness. All too often, the applause that comes with weight loss has very little to do with health or wellbeing, and everything to do with aesthetics. We are praising bodies for becoming smaller – and smaller bodies, in our society, still mean something. They still signal value, worth and control.

But where did we learn that? Where did we learn that thinner equals better; that hunger is something to be proud of; and that taking up less space makes us more lovable? To answer this, we have to go back – back beyond the headlines and the hashtags to the places we first learned how to feel about our bodies. All too often, that starts at home.

The Headlines
- When Ozempic and other GLP-1 drugs burst onto the scene, they thinned bodies and changed the entire cultural narrative about weight, control and health
- These medications quieten food noise and override powerful biological mechanisms that normally make weight loss difficult, which is why they feel life-changing for so many
- Weight-loss injections have exposed the truth that weight is not simply a matter of willpower
- Access is deeply uneven: financial privilege, loosening prescribing practices, drug price increases and a booming black market all continue to shape who gets the drug and how safely they use it
- The rise of these drugs has disrupted the traditional diet industry, pushed global pharmaceutical profits to record highs and blurred the line between healthcare and marketing
- Celebrity influence accelerated the demand for Ozempic and other GLP-1s, somewhat shifting the concept of thinness from aspiration to expectation, and amplifying pressure on everyday people to keep up

A Moment of Reflection
- *What do I believe weight loss will give me, and where did I first learn that those things come from being smaller?*
- *If I've felt pressure to take a GLP-1, was that pressure truly about health, or about fitting in, keeping up with friends, or preventing myself from becoming invisible?*
- *How much compassion do I extend to myself around hunger, appetite and weight, and how much judgement have I absorbed from the culture around me?*
- *What would it mean to make decisions about my body from a place of agency, rather than fear or shame?*

Where Do We Go From Here?

If this chapter highlights anything, it's that the conversation around GLP-1s isn't necessarily about the pharmaceutical drug. Rather it's about the world we've built around bodies – a world that still rewards shrinking and punishes softness, tells us hunger is a failure, that weight is a sign of moral standing and that thinness will grant us social safety.

But naming that system is so powerful. When we understand *why* these drugs feel so compelling, we loosen the grip of shame and stop blaming ourselves for struggling with hunger, or food noise, or weight regain. Seeing our choices in context, rather than in isolation allows us to tap into compassion for ourselves that is so desperately needed.

I don't think the answer from here on out is to either reject GLP-1s or embrace them blindly; I think it's about reclaiming body autonomy in a culture that constantly tries to take it away. It's about asking better questions of the systems that profit from our insecurity and it's about holding a tonne of space for nuance, because these drugs can be life-changing for some and harmful for others, sometimes at the same time.

Most of all, it's about remembering that your worth was never supposed to hang on the size of your body or the number on a scale. The world might feel loud right now with pressure, comparison and noise, but you get to choose whether or not you surrender to it. You can – and should – make any choice you wish, but please, please make sure you do it without shame. Deal?

Chapter 3

Family, Kids and Breaking the Cycle

It Starts At Home...

For millennial and Gen Z women, body image has been shaped by a perfect storm of cultural forces. We grew up in the 1990s and 2000s, an era of toxic tabloid culture, deeply problematic 'makeover' shows and explicit body-shaming. Then came the age of social media: filters, algorithms and an endless scroll of comparison. But while those forces built the environment we grew up in, there's another influence that hit much closer to home: our families, and the people who raised us.

When I refer to 'families', I mean that in the broadest sense – whether that was parents, grandparents, step-parents, carers, older siblings, foster families or any combination of people who shaped our early lives. For some, that environment was nurturing and body-neutral; for others, it was more complicated or even painful. Everyone's story will look different, but these early environments, however they were made up, are often where the seeds of body image are first planted.

Culture sets the standard, of course – it's important we don't forget that, and we'll explore it in greater depth further on in the chapter – but it's often within the four walls of our homes that we learn to internalize certain feelings and ideas about our bodies and our appearances. These beliefs start early on – *really* early on; sometimes before we can even speak – and whether they're intentional or not (usually, they're not) they can leave deep, enduring marks.

This is a difficult topic to discuss for a multitude of reasons. First, I don't think it's helpful to place the blame on our parents for doing the best they could with what they had, and I want this chapter to be respectful of that. I don't want to point fingers or unearth old wounds so that we can stay angry at the past; instead, I want us to understand it. Because how can we break a cycle if we don't fully understand it? Most of our caregivers weren't actively trying to hurt us; they were simply passing down the messages they too had internalized, often from their own upbringings, their own traumas, their own experiences and from a culture that taught them to equate thinness with worth. These patterns are inherited, and I believe that's something really important to keep in mind as we explore this sensitive subject.

That said, it's worth being clear that this compassion isn't an excuse for harm. There's a difference between unintentional conditioning and deliberate cruelty. If you experienced emotional abuse or intentionally harmful behaviour, that pain deserves recognition and care, ideally with the support of a therapist or counsellor.

It's painful to examine this early messaging we were subject to because it asks us to look closely at those we love the most, and the ways they may have helped shape us and our beliefs. It can feel disloyal, or even cruel, to interrogate the dynamics that helped form our body image – especially when our parents or carers were also struggling with their own. I speak to so many women who deeply struggle to reconcile this, but I strongly believe that we can have compassion, love and respect for those who raised us whilst also acknowledging the harm that may have been passed down.

Talking about this subject can also bring up grief. It might mean grieving for the little girl who learned to shrink herself; who thought her body was wrong; who was told not to eat too much bread; or who watched a parent diet constantly or call themselves 'disgusting' in the mirror. It might also prompt grief for the time we've spent at war with ourselves, and grief for what we missed out on while we were preoccupied with trying to be smaller. Despite that, though, I think *not* talking about it is doing ourselves a huge disservice. When we begin to understand where these messages came from, we can start to separate them from who we really are. We can begin to unlearn, start to heal and, if we're raising children ourselves or have young people in our lives, we can hopefully learn to break the cycle for future generations. I really don't want this chapter to be about blame. I want it to focus on clarity and compassion, and I want to give us all the permission to question the stories we were told about our bodies so that we can start writing new ones.

What *is* an Almond Mom Anyway?

The term 'almond mom' exploded on social media a few years ago, inspired by a viral clip of *Real Housewives of Beverly Hills* star Yolanda Hadid and her daughter Gigi. The now-infamous scene saw 19-year-old Gigi calling her mum and complaining of hunger. Yolanda advised her: 'Have a couple of almonds and chew them really well.'

In this brief encounter, Yolanda encapsulated so much of what diet culture represented, and she personified the fatphobia that so many women internalize and, in turn, project onto their own children. The internet exploded with stories: people shared memories of being told to drink water instead of eating; of being taken to a diet group at the age of ten; of being taught to fear fatness at all costs.

An almond mom might count calories obsessively; skip meals; moralise food as 'good' or 'bad'; celebrate thinness, even if it comes at the cost of joy; or constantly talk about her own body in negative terms. She might warn against 'overeating' or push exercise as a means of punishment. These comments might seem subtle: remarks like, 'Are you sure you want seconds?' or 'You look so good, have you lost weight?' or 'I can't eat that, I was bad yesterday.' When you hear them over and over, though, these innocuous-seeming comments can start to shape your internal narrative – especially coming from someone you love and trust, and who acts as your reference point for how to move through the world.

A parent's words hold weight, especially when they're talking about something as personal and vulnerable as our bodies. When a caregiver expresses fear around food or disgust towards their own appearance, it's inevitable that you might internalize the message that bodies are problems to be solved, and hunger is something to suppress. For so many of us, food wasn't just food – it was morality, too. It was reward and punishment; something to be earned or restricted. We were taught to associate hunger with success and fullness with failure. We learnt to suck in our stomachs, scan our reflections in the mirror for flaws, and to believe that gaining weight was the worst thing that could happen. Often, it was through our mothers that we first witnessed these behaviours.

Despite this, though, I'm not sure 'almond mom' is a particularly helpful term. It feels somehow flippant, almost mocking, and it oversimplifies something that is actually deeply complex and often painful. Behind every 'almond mom' is a woman who was once a child herself, often raised on the same messages, the same body rules, the same fear of taking up space. She no doubt had an 'almond mom' too. It was all completely misguided, of course, and the results were damaging, but so much of what many of our mums were trying to do was help us 'fit in', to protect us from criticism by teaching us to criticize ourselves first. All too often they attempted to shield us from a fatphobic world by trying to shape us into its ideal. In most cases, they weren't trying to hurt us; they just genuinely believed that being smaller was better and they wanted the best for us. It doesn't make it right, of course, but it does make it more understandable.

Another reason I find the term 'almond mom' unhelpful is that it's not only mums who exhibit these types of behaviours. It's true, and important to acknowledge, that the maternal role is pivotal in a child's development, particularly for girls – mothers are often our very first mirror: we observe how they look at themselves, how they talk about their bodies, how they navigate food and exercise, and we absorb those cues long before we actually understand them. That influence is powerful, and it matters. But diet culture isn't *just* passed down from mother to daughter.

'I think it's unfair to place the pressure squarely on mothers' shoulders,' says Molly Forbes, campaigner, speaker and author of *Body Happy Kids*. 'It lets dads and other important adult roles in a child's life off the hook.'

When we only talk about 'almond moms' and the influence of mothers, we risk creating a narrative where women are solely responsible for the harm, and men are merely bystanders in their children's lives. 'When we focus solely on mothers, we reinforce this idea that they are the gatekeepers of body image, and that's both inaccurate and unfair,' says Molly. 'It loads them with even more pressure in a system that's already stacked against them. Meanwhile, it allows other influential figures to opt out of responsibility altogether. But body image isn't just a "mum issue", it's a culture-wide issue and everyone has a part to play.'

The Role of Family as a Whole

Dads can play a huge role in shaping body image – sometimes in overt ways, like commenting on our weight, and sometimes in more subtle, loaded ways, like teasing us about food or praising thinness in women. A throwaway comment at the dinner table or a joke about someone's body on TV can lodge itself deep when it comes from someone you look up to. I had a pretty surreal experience with my own dad a couple of years ago – one I will never forget. For some context: his nickname for me when I was younger was 'pretty but plump'. It was said with affection, but it quietly confirmed a belief I had already formed about myself: I could only be truly beautiful, without any 'buts', if I was thin. As a girl growing up in a world that dictates beauty as a woman's currency, this was a painful but crystal-clear conclusion to draw. I had to be thin, and if I wasn't, my body was always going to be a 'but'.

Then, when I was doing the Q&A section of a panel talk in 2023 on body image and generational influence, my dad, who was in the audience, stood up and signalled that he'd like to speak. My heart raced as he waited for the microphone, and I wondered what on earth he was going to say to this room full of strangers. 'I just want to say sorry for the impact me and your mum might have had on you growing up,' he started, and my eyes immediately began to fill with tears. 'I know that there's lots of things I said and didn't say that will have made you feel the way you do about your body, and I'm sorry.'

I fought hard not to *properly* cry, but this moment meant a lot to me. It was healing – not so much the apology, I don't think, but his acknowledgement and recognition that his words and his actions had impacted me. It felt really brave of him to face the cognitive dissonance that comes with admitting you've been wrong, and accepting you may have caused harm – especially in front of a room full of strangers. After the talk, several women came up to me in tears. They told me they hadn't expected to cry, but when my dad stood up and apologized, it cracked something open for them. It didn't heal the relationship with their own parents, of course, but it gave them a sense of validation that they had been craving.

It's difficult to unpack the harm that can come from those closest to us: it often feels quiet or subtle, and wrapped up alongside care and good intentions, which can leave you doubting yourself. *Was I too sensitive? Did I imagine it?* But watching a father publicly acknowledge that words *do* matter made many of those women feel seen.

It's not just our parents who impact our body image, though – it's also our siblings, aunties, uncles, grandparents, family friends, our teachers. So often, the onus is placed solely on mothers, but children absorb messages from *everyone* around them. Every comment, whether it's about someone else's weight, what's on their plate, how they look in a certain outfit, or a passing judgement about someone else's body, gets stored and contributes to beliefs around what's desirable, what's acceptable and what's worthy.

I recall in perfect detail one Sunday when I was a young – and hungry! – teenager, sitting at the dinner table, halfway through my roast dinner when a distant relative said to my mum and dad: 'She puts it away this one, doesn't she?!' Everyone laughed, except me. My cheeks burned red, I pinched my thigh to try and stop myself crying, and I discreetly put down my knife and fork, making a quiet promise to myself to eat less. Another example that's seared into my memory is hearing my grandad say that hugging me was 'like hugging a teddy bear' because I was 'so chubby'. I was sixteen and absolutely mortified. Twenty years later, I've still not forgotten that comment.

The commentary wasn't just aimed at me, either. I grew up with four sisters, and whilst I know that isn't everyone's experience, what is devastatingly common is the constant comparison that happens between siblings. In every family with multiple kids, it's almost inevitable that certain roles are assigned: the smart one, the funny one, the sporty one, the thin one. That last one may go unsaid, but it is very often made very clear: from the way adults compliment one sister's figure and stay silent on yours; in the way family photos are scrutinized with comments like, 'you've got a much rounder face than your sister'; or how one of you is encouraged to finish her plate while another's eating is subtly policed. These dynamics are rarely intentional, but they cut deep – especially when your body feels like your defining trait. In a house full of girls, I learned very early on that bodies are currency, and that thinness carries the highest value.

All this constant commentary and subtle messaging plants something else in you too: the belief that your body is always being measured – not *just* against a cultural ideal, but against the people closest to you in the world. One of the hardest things in this aspect – and this is honestly quite hard for me to admit – was watching how people responded when one of my sisters lost weight. There was so much excitement, a whole new load of approval and endless praise. 'You look AMAZING!' they'd gush. They didn't mean harm – they probably thought they were being kind – but I absorbed the interactions. I noticed, firstly, how the compliments would change my sister's posture, her smile, her confidence. I also noticed how *I* felt at these words: like it would take losing weight for me to be accepted and approved of and praised, too. It wasn't jealousy, exactly – I think it was a more confusing tangle of feelings like guilt, shame and comparison. I didn't want my sister to feel any less joy, but I couldn't help feeling less seen.

I sent my sisters these paragraphs after I wrote them to ask what they thought. One replied: 'God, I felt that too. And I hated those compliments for myself . . . They made me feel good for a second but then made me realize that people were watching my body closely, and that's a horrible feeling.'

Another said: 'I always noticed who got complimented and who didn't. When it was to someone else, the silence about my own body felt loud. It made me wonder what people thought when they looked at me, and the sentiment behind their words was clear: you should do the same, you'd look better, you'd be praised too.'

Another sister had a different take: 'I was more scared about negative comments. We could always sense the disapproval after gaining weight – even if nothing was said, the pity seemed to hang in the air and we'd often be asked if we were "on a diet". I was so terrified about the negative comments that I would ask my mum to warn people ahead of seeing them again that I'd gained weight. It felt like a way of anticipating and controlling the situation.'

Reading their replies broke my heart a little. From such a young age, we were so painfully aware of how people were perceiving our bodies. We'd learned to anticipate it and to even try to pre-empt the disappointment in a room. All of this, understandably, had an impact on our eating. In various ways, we all struggled with disordered eating, and some of us with eating disorders. I know this will be the case for so many of you, too: when we're growing up, we're like little sponges, which means that we're extremely absorbent to the factors around us, often learning from the older people around us that thinness could be equated with safety; that losing weight, no matter the means, could earn you praise, whilst gaining weight would earn you concern or, worse, disappointment. As a result, of course, we adapted: we focused on shrinking; we obsessed; we restricted; and we tried to control what we could in a world that was trying to shape us.

It's no wonder that so many of us carry complicated

relationships with food, exercise and our bodies – because when love and acceptance feel even slightly tied to how you look, eating becomes your way to control that.

All the comments and comparisons leave a mark, and it's totally fair and understandable to feel angry and hurt in moments like that – I know I certainly did. But with time and distance, I've also come to understand that those comments didn't come from nowhere. Those adults were shaped by the culture that they grew up in – a culture that was, in many ways, even more brutal than the one I came of age in.

The Not-Too-Distant History of Diet Culture

To get a better idea of what it was like for the older generations growing up, we need to acknowledge that the generation that raised us was sold diet culture with a capital D. They were the era of phrases like, 'a moment on the lips, a lifetime on the hips' and 'if you can pinch more than an inch . . .'. Tabloid body-shaming was the norm; they lived through the rise of low-fat *everything* and weekly Weight Watchers meetings were just another part of life. Adverts for diet products were in abundance during the 1960s and 1970s, and they were overwhelmingly targeted at women.

During my research for this chapter, I trawled through hundreds of vintage diet ads and saw less than a handful that featured men. When they did appear, they weren't the target of the ad; rather, they were featured as the prize for thinness. The overrepresentation of women was glaring, but even more insidious was how many of these ads were tapping into women's insecurities about being attractive to men. One ad promoting Metrecal, which was a bright, almost neon-pink – think Pepto-Bismol – and essentially a meal-replacement protein shake, showed a thin woman standing in front of a log fire, staring lovingly at a male partner. The caption reads: 'How slender you were in the glow of the fire... Would he think so now?' before encouraging readers to buy Metrecal, which, incidentally, was pulled from shelves in the late 1970s, after being linked to deaths. Another from SEGO Diet Food used almost the same script: a woman in a swimsuit beside her fully clothed husband, the line: *'Your honeymoon figure... How slender it was. Would he think so now?'*

Basically, your worth as a woman and your partner's affection for you were being framed as conditional on maintaining a youthful, 'slender' body. Big sigh.

What's especially striking, though, is how these ads resisted the social climate of the time. The 1960s and 1970s were decades of enormous change for women, with women entering the workforce in larger numbers, demanding reproductive rights, beginning to push back against rigid gender roles. But as women's power and independence grew, the diet industry doubled down. It reminded women that even if they could be successful and intelligent and free, none of it would even matter unless they were also thin.

Another ad that stopped me in my tracks was a 1970s advert for a product called Shape – a diet drink marketed specifically at women. The image shows three women on a beach all posing together: two are wearing bikinis and one is wearing a jumper. The headline alone tells you everything you need to know about the tone: 'You know why she's wearing the sweatshirt, don't you?' *Eurgh!* The implication is immediate and brutal: she's overweight, she's ashamed, and we're all in on the joke. The jumper is a symbol of failure. Then, of course, comes the 'solution': a product to help you 'stop eating'. The sting is made worse by the fact that the woman pictured wearing the sweatshirt is, by any standard, already thin. I'm not even paraphrasing here: it literally says, 'Face it, you've got to stop eating', in bold. Further down, they say Shape 'tastes good enough to help you stop eating'.

It didn't stop there: ads from this era also leaned heavily on pseudo-science. Laxatives were marketed as everyday wellness tools and appetite suppressants were packaged as cheerful lifestyle aids, promoted in daytime TV slots with women happily proclaiming that they 'didn't feel hungry anymore'. One popular ad for an over-the-counter diet pill called Obetrol in the 1960s and early 1970s promised that users could 'eat anything and still lose weight' thanks to its magical fat-absorbing powders. Obetrol was, essentially, amphetamine, or speed. The focus was on rapid, visible results with little to no regard for the side effects.

Weight-loss ads from the 1980s were less explicit in their misogyny – they no longer told women outright that they had to lose weight to be attractive to men – but they were still *rife* with diet culture. 'NOW! Lose 10 pounds FAST', reads one advert for Carnation, a diet shake, alongside a photo of a woman in a swimsuit. 'Losing weight is delicious with SlimFast', reads another, accompanied by a photo of a woman also in a swimsuit. Diet Coke launched in the early 1980s, and was marketed heavily to weight-conscious consumers, especially women. 'The real cola taste with just one calorie', read one of their ads, 'for looking good and feeling good'. The tagline was accompanied by – you guessed it! – a woman in a swimsuit. Chitosan-based 'fat-binding' pills surged in popularity during the 1980s: these products claimed they could absorb up to 60 per cent of the fat in your food, effectively letting you eat whatever you wanted while still losing weight. The science behind it was sketchy at best and there appears to have been no solid evidence behind these claims, but the marketing went all in, and the ads were so persuasive, the culture so desperate, that the product didn't actually have to work. They just needed to sell hope. The 1980s also saw Weight Watchers reach an all-time high subscriber count; new diet giant Jenny Craig entered the market; Jane Fonda's famous workout VHS tapes sold millions; and, of course, we had that infamous moment when Oprah dragged a wagon containing 67 lb of animal fat onstage, as we discussed in the previous chapter.

It's hard to say for sure, but arguably the 1990s were even more toxic: the weight-loss industry was thriving, with a reported value of $51 billion, and diets like Atkins were enjoying an enormously popular resurgence. This period was also synonymous with 'heroin chic', a super-skinny aesthetic associated with the decade's most famous model, Kate Moss. Celebrity workout VHS tapes were everywhere, like Cindy Crawford's *Shape Your Body Workout*, and sales were booming in the early 1990s.

Throughout these decades, magazines were filled with tips like drinking vinegar before meals to 'cut cravings', chewing gum to distract yourself from hunger, and eating ice cubes to burn calories. These ideas weren't fringe ideas or some kind of 'alternative thinking' – they were part of the mainstream conversation around health, weight and simply being a woman. Essentially, you couldn't open a magazine, switch on the TV, or even go food shopping without being told, subtly or overtly, that your body wasn't good enough.

By the late 1970s and 1980s, fat itself had become the enemy. 'Low-fat' became the buzzword of the era and supermarket shelves were bursting with 'lite', 'fat-free' and 'diet' products: yoghurts, salad dressings, cheese slices, biscuits. Fat, a vital macronutrient, was rebranded as something shameful that ought to be avoided at all costs. The obsession with 'low-fat' ran so deep that it would shape the way women ate for decades to come.

The fitness industry was riddled with diet culture, too: exercising wasn't about building strength, doing something you enjoyed or that might give you more energy; rather the focus was on burning calories, getting your 'bikini body' and toning and sculpting.

I could go on – and on, and on, because there are literally thousands of examples – but I think you get the point: older generations were surrounded by these messages, and through them women were told what to buy, what to do and who to be. Some adverts told women to lose weight, while others encouraged them to gain 'curves' to have a 'more womanly' physique, but either way, all these ads emphasised the need for self-control and self-discipline in women and made clear that their worth would be measured through their body size. They were continually demanded to conform to a set of body ideals and, inevitably, many of the women who raised us will unfortunately have been victims of this.

Given the culture that preceded our own, it therefore feels vital that we understand the context in which older family members – especially mothers – grew up when we think about the way their behaviours have impacted us. All too many parents passed on the knowledge that they had, teaching us the same rules that had been drilled into them. What else were they – and their mothers – supposed to teach us if not the stuff they knew? It's clear that they had internalized the knowledge that life would be easier to navigate if you were thinner; you would be more desirable to men if you were thinner; you'd be happier if you were thinner; and you'd be the best version of yourself if you were, you guessed it . . . thinner.

It is my firm belief that body obsession is passed down through generations not because women want to harm their daughters, but because they believe it's the only way to keep them safe. If we look at Yolanda Hadid, the original 'almond mom', as an example of this, her behaviour starts to make more sense. This is a woman who spent her youth working as a model, a famously brutal industry where thinness is not just glorified but enforced. As she aged (a cardinal sin for a woman and especially in the modelling world) and had children (another act often perceived as career suicide), she watched her own career gradually fade. So, when her daughters – young, beautiful, and full of the potential the industry prizes – braced themselves to step into the modelling world, it feels almost inevitable that Yolanda would pass onto them the 'rules' she was taught. I have no doubt that, in her mind, that comment about the almonds wasn't one of cruelty, but rather an attempt at being helpful by preparing them, and teaching them what it would take to succeed.

I'm aware that I am projecting my own assumptions onto Yolanda here, and I may be way off the mark, but I do think it's worth exploring what might be going on beneath the surface. This is how these cycles work: they're rarely driven by malice, but rather by deeply internalized beliefs about what makes a woman valuable.

I'm also aware that I'm really pressing on the point of not assigning blame, and that's intentional, because I believe that blame is counterproductive and keeps us stuck. It locks us into binary thinking – right and wrong, good and bad – but this conversation demands more complexity. I'm in no way trying to excuse harmful behaviours, but I also think it's about having a greater understanding so that we ourselves can heal, move forward and begin to break the cycle. When we shift from blame to curiosity, we make way for compassion – not just for our mothers, or other family members or external influences, but for ourselves, too.

So, How Can We Break These Patterns?

I spoke to Phillippa Diedrichs, research psychologist and body image and mental health expert, to gain a better insight into what we can do to break the cycle. 'I think taking a step back to think about why someone is doing what they're doing and what pressures they've been exposed to might create a bit of a buffer between the intensity of your emotions to that person,' she says. Although Phillippa believes compassion is important, and that carrying blame and resentment for someone isn't necessarily a healthy path forward, she notes that boundaries are also key. 'You can be compassionate, but you can also set healthy boundaries to protect your own mental health.

'You can be clear in that you don't want to discuss weight or dieting or express discomfort when your appearance is commented on, and if those boundaries are crossed, you're well within your rights to remove yourself from that situation,' adds Phillippa. 'So, I think compassion and accountability can exist simultaneously.'

This point about the possibility of compassion and accountability coexisting is so important, and I want to explore it a little further. The idea of having compassion for our family or loved ones might make you assume that it means accepting everything they say, tolerating uncomfortable comments, maintaining a happy smile and keeping quiet so as not to rock the boat. But *real* compassion, both for others and for ourselves, often looks like choosing discomfort over silence. Confrontation can be so difficult, but what's more important is protecting our peace, our progress and our healing. Boundaries can be one of the most loving things we can do for all people involved, and they don't have to be angry or unkind (unless that's how you feel they have to be, and of course that's valid and absolutely your prerogative). They can be kind and calm but also firm.

So, how on earth do we go about doing that? What does it look like on a practical level?

Here are a few compassionate ways we might enforce boundaries around body talk, food policing or weight commentary – whether it's with a parent, a grandparent, a sibling, an aunty, uncle, family friend, or anyone else:

Use 'I' statements
These are simple but powerful. We're not attacking the person making the comment, instead we're sharing how something affects us. For example:
- 'I'm working really hard on having a better relationship with food and my body, and comments about dieting make that harder for me. Please can we keep the conversation away from those topics?'
- 'I'd appreciate if we didn't talk about food in a judgemental way – it's something I'm working on for myself.'

Have a conversation about your boundaries beforehand
If we know we're heading into a potentially triggering situation like a family meal, holiday gathering, or a wedding, it could be helpful to pre-empt any uncomfortable situations – a text or phone call ahead of time can be really helpful in making sure these comments or topics don't come up:
- 'I just wanted to flag that I'm trying not to talk about bodies, weight or diets at the moment – it's something that I'm working on, and I'd really love and appreciate your support.'

Redirecting
If someone slips up – and this is likely, given how ingrained these beliefs and behaviours are – we can gently redirect:
- 'I know you don't mean any harm by that comment, but it's not helpful for me right now. Can we change the subject?'
- 'Let's not go down the food/body talk road – tell me about your week instead!'

Walk away if necessary
As Phillippa advised, sometimes the kindest thing we can do is to remove ourselves from the situation. We don't need to stay in conversations or environments that feel unsafe – especially if our boundaries are being repeatedly ignored. Here's how this might look:
- 'I'm going to take a break from this conversation; I'll come back when I feel more comfortable.'

- 'I love you, but I'm not willing to keep having this same conversation. Let's talk when we can focus on something else.'

I know that for many of us, especially the people pleasers among us (Hi!), setting boundaries with family feels incredibly hard – it can bring up guilt, fear of rejection, fear of hurting someone's feelings or being seen as 'difficult'. But I need you to know that your healing matters, and stating these boundaries and having them respected is not in any way unreasonable. You are asking for what you need and it's your right to do so.

One thing I find really helpful to remember when setting boundaries is that, when we approach them from a place of self-respect and calm, rather than shame and anger, we're not preventing connection – we're actually creating the conditions for healthier connections to exist, and even flourish.

Reparenting Ourselves and Changing the Narrative

Once we begin setting boundaries with the outside world, we're often left face-to-face with the internalized voices we've absorbed over the years. Even when the comments from others stop, we likely still hear echoes of them in our own self-talk: 'don't eat that', 'suck in your stomach', 'you don't need such a big portion', 'why can't you be more disciplined?'.

As Professor Jane Ogden explains, 'From the moment we are born, we learn about the many meanings of food, our relationship to food and our own bodies. This can result in body talk that is often critical. These are very ingrained and often without our full awareness. They're also attached to many triggers in our external worlds (people, situations) and emotional worlds (thoughts and emotions). Even when we are aware of them, these many triggers can generate them, which can feel uncomfortable.'

This part requires work, but one of the most empowering parts of healing is the realization that we can learn to reparent ourselves and silence that inner critic. The validation we craved from our parents; the safety we never got to feel in our own bodies; the forgiveness we needed – that can all come from us. It might not erase what has happened in the past, but it empowers us to move forward in a kinder and more compassionate manner and speak to the small child inside of us who believed that she had to earn love by being smaller.

Reparenting is essentially a way of meeting the needs that weren't met in childhood. If our caregivers were unable to provide body neutrality, freedom around food, or a healthy relationship with an inevitably changing body, we now have the opportunity to give those things to ourselves. As Jane says, the first step is recognition: 'being reflective and keeping a record of any internal dialogue together with the triggers.' From there, the shift from self-criticism to self-compassion involves 'facing this dialogue, talking about it with others, thinking where it has come from, looking for evidence to contradict it, practising an inner dialogue to refute any negativity and sharing these rebuttals with others.'

This process, just like all important and meaningful work, isn't easy, but Jane assures us that it is possible. What she's describing is the slow unpicking of habits that were never really ours to begin with – the internalized rules about food, worth and control that we absorbed simply through watching and listening. For many of us, these manifest as a cruel inner critic that comes out when we're tired, stressed or standing in front of the mirror.

Reparenting interrupts that cycle. It's about catching ourselves in the moment we tell ourselves, 'You don't need that second helping' and asking instead, 'What do I *actually* need right now?' Sometimes the answer IS food, and sometimes it's comfort, rest, reassurance or emotional support. The same goes for comments like 'You look awful today' or 'You shouldn't wear that' – the question becomes, 'Where does this come from and what am I really feeling?'

This kind of self-enquiry doesn't come naturally to people who grew up in an environment steeped in criticism. When that critical voice has lived inside us for years, perhaps disguised as discipline or as humour, it can be hard to recognize it for what it really is. It takes practice, and it's tough, but over time it builds a new language – one rooted in curiosity rather than criticism.

Jane's emphasis on recognition and reflection is key here. Keeping a record of our internal dialogue sounds a bit odd, but it's surprisingly revealing. Writing down when the voice appears, what triggered it, and what emotion it brings up can help us see patterns that were previously invisible. Often, the harshest self-talk flares up when other things are happening in our lives: maybe work is overwhelming, a relationship feels strained or we're struggling with a big life event. The voice about food or weight can sometimes be about neither of those two things; rather, it's about control. Seeing that clearly can help to loosen its grip.

From there, the practice of gentle rebuttal – talking back to that voice – is transformative. It can be as simple as saying, 'That's the old story. I don't believe that anymore'. You could also imagine yourself speaking to your younger self, who only wanted to feel safe and accepted. Each time you respond with empathy rather than shame, you rewire the association between self-criticism and safety. Over time, that compassion starts to feel more instinctive than punishment.

And, equally as important: sharing these inner dialogues with others helps dismantle their power. Shame thrives in secrecy and when we talk about our food guilt, our body worries or the inherited scripts we still struggle with, we find that so, so many of us are fighting the same battle! That collective recognition doesn't, of course, erase the damage or immediately 'fix' us, but it does remind us that the voices aren't personal failings.

All of this, ultimately, is the act of reparenting: choosing, over and over again, to replace punishment with compassion and understanding and control with care. We have to show that inner critic that it no longer runs the show.

Breaking the Cycle with The Young People in Our Lives

If we are raising children of our own, or spending time with nieces, nephews, or our friends' kids, we have an incredible opportunity. We can finally start to break the cycle and do our best to ensure that the next generation don't grow up plagued by body image doubts and a preoccupation with eating. We have an opportunity to rewrite the narrative. Of course, this doesn't mean we'll get everything right, by any means, but it does mean that we can try, and we can use our curiosity, honesty and self-compassion to foster a better environment for our kids than the one we grew up in.

So, how *do* we go about breaking the cycle? It starts with unlearning our own patterns of behaviour. Diet culture is woven so tightly into the fabric of our society that many of us don't even realize how often it shows up in our day-to-day lives. It's hidden in compliments that seem harmless ('You look amazing – have you lost weight?'), in the way we talk about 'earning' a 'treat' or in off-the-cuff comments about 'being good' for skipping dessert. Kids are *always* listening to and taking in what the adults around them say.

This isn't confined to food and body talk, either: even the ways we speak to children can reinforce those same old patterns of appearance-based validation. Little girls are often praised for being 'pretty' or told how 'cute' their outfit is, while little boys are called 'brave', 'strong' or 'clever'. It's subtle, but it plants a seed that girls are valued for how they look, and boys for what they do. Breaking that cycle isn't about never giving a compliment again, it's about broadening what we notice and what we celebrate. Instead of focusing on appearance, we can praise curiosity, kindness, creativity, strength, humour, effort or bravery.

'I feel like it's really important to remember there isn't necessarily a right or wrong way to unlearn this stuff,' says Molly Forbes, campaigner, speaker and author of *Body Happy Kids*. 'Diet culture thrives on shame and making us feel less than – if we take those same feelings into unlearning it, we're just substituting one thing that makes us feel rubbish for something else. There's a difference between *recognizing* harmful patterns and holding ourselves accountable to do better and drenching ourselves with shame when we inevitably fall back into our feedback loops about bodies and worth. If we're not careful, we can end up feeling like we're either failing at having the 'right' body or failing at feeling the 'right' way about that body.

'It's exhausting – and toxic positivity isn't going to help our kids learn a more compassionate approach for themselves, either. It's hard being a human and having a body in the culture we live in. Even just remembering that can be validating – both for us and the kids in our lives.'

The first step is awareness: noticing the way these messages live in our language, our habits and our behaviour. Because the reality is that kids don't learn how to relate to their bodies just from what we say, they *absorb* what we model. They see how we look at ourselves in the mirror, they hear the frustration in our voices when clothes feel tight and they notice when we skip meals, restrict certain foods or use exercise as punishment. Even a subtle sigh or a self-deprecating joke about our appearance can send a message.

That's why one of the most powerful ways to break the cycle is by becoming more mindful of how we speak and act about our own bodies and food. This includes how we talk about other people's bodies, too: no matter how well-intentioned, body-based comments reinforce the idea that appearance is what matters most. When we remove body commentary altogether, we create space for our kids to focus on other, far more meaningful aspects of themselves and others.

We can also begin to shift the narrative through how we speak about food and movement. So much of diet culture teaches us to moralise food – labelling things as 'good' or 'bad', 'clean' or 'junk', 'naughty' or 'healthy' – but this language shapes not only how we view food but how we view ourselves in relation to it. It ties our worth to what we're consuming.

Instead, we can focus on how food makes us feel: energised, satisfied, comforted, connected... We can talk about how different foods serve different purposes: some give us quick energy, some keep us full for longer, some are nostalgic, some are celebratory, and some are social. And *all* of them are allowed. All have value – and by removing shame and moral judgement from food, we create space for children to listen to their own hunger and fullness cues, to trust their bodies and to develop a relationship with food that is intuitive and free from fear.

This also means letting go of strict rules and embracing a more relaxed, balanced approach to eating. It's OK to eat vegetables *and* cake. It's OK to have seconds. It's OK to eat emotionally sometimes. When we model that ease around food, our children learn that eating doesn't have to come with anxiety, guilt or control.

Exercise, meanwhile, can be approached with a similar mindset. Rather than framing movement as something we *have* to do to 'burn off' food or change our bodies, we can talk about it as something we *get* to do – a privilege, and a way to feel strong, joyful, energised or calm. We can model movement as a tool for mental health and for fun, rather than a punishment.

Just as important is the way we approach rest: in a culture that idolize productivity and often links thinness to discipline, rest is often framed as laziness or weakness. But rest is vital – and when we honour it in our own lives, we give our children permission to honour their needs, too. Whether it's taking a break, listening to our bodies or simply not forcing activity when exhausted, these are essential lessons in self-respect and body trust.

The way we speak about clothing and body changes also

matters. Children's bodies are constantly changing, and when they inevitably outgrow their clothes, it should never be framed as a problem. Instead of showing any kind of negative feelings about a size increase, we can respond neutrally: 'Your body's growing, let's get you clothes that feel good and fit you well.' This normalizes growth, rather than pathologizing it.

Praise can be another place of transformation. Instead of complimenting appearance, we can praise effort, creativity, strength or kindness. Instead of 'you look pretty', we can say 'you seem really happy today'. We can celebrate our children's bodies not for how they look, but what they can do. Over time, this helps them internalize a sense of self-worth that doesn't hinge on external validation or physical ideals.

I am very aware that all the above is a big ask for those of us (which is most of us!) who have grown up steeped in diet culture. So many habits are deeply ingrained in us. Many of us were praised for shrinking, rewarded for restriction and shown – whether it was directly or indirectly – that the way our bodies looked was a marker for how lovable, successful or valuable we were. So, to begin unlearning that conditioning, all while trying to raise children in a different, more positive way, is no small feat.

But we don't have to be perfect to make a difference. As Molly says, this work isn't about getting everything right – that's likely impossible. But we can be willing to try; willing to notice; to pause before we say something; to make amends when we slip up. Every time we choose a more compassionate response, either towards ourselves or our children, we're planting the seeds for something . . . better.

When we do slip back into old patterns – whether that's criticizing our own reflections or defaulting to body-based commentary – we can name it and attempt to repair it. 'That wasn't helpful. I'm still working on speaking more kindly to myself,' might be a good response. These moments of honesty are so powerful – because they show our children that growth isn't about perfection but rather about awareness and the courage to keep learning.

We can also take small but meaningful steps to reshape the media and messages we (and our children) are exposed to. We can curate our feed to include diverse, joyful representations of bodies, follow fat-positive and anti-diet creators, educators, and artists and seek out books and content that promote body respect, food neutrality, and self-compassion. The more we engage with content that reflects our values, the more those values become embedded in our everyday lives.

Since I began this work, I've thought a lot about how I'll talk to my son Tommy about bodies and food. I've been lucky enough to spend years consistently unlearning the damage of diet culture and those beliefs no longer feel like my default, and that might make it easier. I have worked so hard to reshape my language and beliefs about my body and food, but I know I am bound to have blind spots, and I wouldn't be surprised if some of them show up in parenthood.

Ultimately though, as Molly said, the goal isn't to be perfect but to be conscious. To try really hard, and to course-correct whenever we mess up. I want Tommy to live his life not just feeling neutral about his own body but also understanding the world he's growing up in – and the pressures that women, in particular, face. I want him to recognize how unfairly bodies are policed and judged, how much time and energy women are taught to spend on shrinking themselves, and how deeply these messages can hurt.

Above all, I want him to meet that understanding with kindness and compassion – to be someone who never makes another person feel bad about their appearance, who doesn't comment on bodies, and who values people for *who* they are, rather than *how* they look. That, to me, is one of the most powerful legacies I could hope to pass on.

That's the kind of ripple effect that this work can have. It doesn't stop with us. It extends outwards: to our children, our communities, and the next generation, and this is why it matters so much.

So yes, our parents had a huge impact. And no, they didn't get everything right. But in most cases, they were trying – and now we get to try too. We get to choose what we carry forward and what we leave behind.

The Headlines

- Our earliest ideas about food, bodies and worth are shaped long before we're aware of them; they're often picked up in the ordinary moments of family life
- Harmful body beliefs usually aren't born from malice; they're inherited through generations of diet culture, patriarchy and impossible beauty standards
- Parents, especially mothers, absorbed deeply damaging cultural messaging about discipline, thinness and desirability, and unintentionally passed that language on
- Body image is shaped not just by mothers, but by fathers, siblings, grandparents, teachers and any adult who comments on bodies, food or appearance
- Even subtle remarks, comparisons and 'jokes' can shape a child's belief about their body
- Breaking the cycle requires awareness, boundaries and self-compassion, not perfection
- Reparenting ourselves is a powerful part of the healing process: noticing our internalized scripts, challenging them and creating a more compassionate inner voice
- We can raise the next generation with less shame, more ease around food and a deeper sense of body trust

A Moment of Reflection
- *What are the earliest memories I have of hearing adults talk about bodies, food or weight?*
- *Which messages from childhood still show up in my inner voice today?*
- *Where do I notice myself repeating patterns I've inherited, and where do I feel the urge to do things differently?*
- *How much of my self-talk is actually my own, and how much is an echo of someone else's fear, shame or insecurity?*
- *When I imagine raising children or influencing young people, what do I want them to learn about bodies, hunger, pleasure and worth?*
- *What boundaries do I need to protect my healing, even if they feel uncomfortable to set with people I love?*
- *If I could speak to the younger version of myself, what reassurance would she have needed most?*

Where Do We Go From Here?

When we choose curiosity instead of shame, boundaries instead of silence, compassion instead of criticism, we create something our younger selves never had – safety. And that safety is what allows children to grow into adults who trust their bodies, honour their hunger, and move through the world without believing their worth is tied to a number, a size or a reflection.

This is how cycles broken: gently, consistently and with a huge dose of awareness and compassion. Our parents shaped us with the tools they had; now we get to choose different ones. And when we do, the impact ripples outward – it reaches our children, our nieces and nephews, our students, our communities.

The patterns that shaped us were powerful, yes, but they are not permanent, and the best thing we can offer the next generation isn't thinness but a chance to live without the fear of not being enough just as we are.

Chapter 4

Pregnancy and Postpartum

No one really prepares you for what happens to your body during pregnancy and birth. They'll talk about stretch marks or tiredness, maybe even mention doing pelvic floor exercises, but it's very rare that anyone talks about what it feels like to wake up in a body that you don't recognize anymore.

My Pregnancy Story

Pregnancy was a wild ride for me when it came to body image. I had no idea what to expect, but if I'm being honest, I thought I'd be fine. I work in this space, I talk about body image all the time, I've done a lot of unlearning of unhealthy thought patterns and behaviours, so I sort of assumed that I'd sail through it unfazed . . . right?! And in the beginning, I did. My first trimester passed with little change in how I felt about the way my body looked. I was exhausted – my God, that tiredness is something else – and I felt queasy, yes, but I remained relatively body-neutral and more preoccupied with scans, injections and pessaries (the joys of IVF!).

Then came the second trimester, which was a real curveball – but maybe not in the way you might imagine. As my bump began to bloom, so did my confidence in my body. My body was growing, changing, expanding – and for the first time in my life, those changes were met not with judgement or silence or pity, but with awe and admiration. Strangers smiled at me, friends complimented me. The narrative around my body had shifted to something overwhelmingly positive, and I have to admit that it felt intoxicating. It was as if I had suddenly been granted permission to take up space – finally. I wore tight dresses and proudly showed off my bump, and I *celebrated* my body in a way I just never had before.

But the positivity I felt for my body transcended how it looked: I was in awe of what my body could do. Every scan, every kick I felt, every change in shape felt like proof that my body was something to admire and appreciate. There's something bittersweet about that, because it shouldn't take growing another human being to feel proud of your body. Yet, for so many of us, that's the first time we're told our changing bodies are beautiful – the irony being that they're changing for someone else.

Prior to pregnancy, all my therapy and body image work had seen me arrive in a space where I felt neutral about my body, but I had never actively *celebrated* it. For someone who had spent so much of her life desperately avoiding mirrors and hiding in oversized, baggy clothing, this was unfamiliar but glorious territory. Finding immense relief and joy in softness, I was witnessing my body do something extraordinary – and the world seemed to agree.

Unfortunately, that golden window didn't last: the third trimester hit me like a tonne of bricks. My body kept growing, but it also started to swell. I developed a remarkable amount of fluid retention, to the point where I had to get my rings cut off my fingers and wear my husband Dave's shoes because mine wouldn't fit. The area around my eyes was so swollen that I had to start each day with my face in a bowl of ice water for a bit of comfort and I couldn't wear socks at all – which wasn't exactly ideal in the depths of winter!

Slowly, I felt things changing. Some of the compliments began to be replaced with concern and I distinctly remember someone telling me I looked 'really puffy'. This, combined with the sheer effort of simply *being* in my body whilst feeling so physically uncomfortable was all just . . . a lot. I couldn't move like I had before pregnancy – even getting up a flight of stairs was a gargantuan effort. I couldn't sleep, and I didn't recognize my reflection anymore. The body confidence I'd felt in the second trimester waned and I felt increasingly self-conscious.

Then I gave birth via an elective C-section to a little boy we named Tommy. One minute I was looking at my bump in the mirror, and the next I was holding this tiny, perfect little human – all while feeling like I'd been hit by a truck. Even though my C-section was planned, nothing really prepares you for the feeling of being so completely out of control of your body: you're awake but detached from your own experience while things are happening *to* you rather than *with* you. Yet, strangely, I also felt safe in the hands of medical professionals and there was a quiet power in surrendering (unfamiliar territory for a self-confessed control freak!).

There was such an intense amount of love when Tommy was born, but also a profound feeling of shock. I remember standing in the shower the day after giving birth and sobbing. I was no longer carrying Tommy inside me, and my body felt empty and hollow. Even though he was in the room next to me, I felt a deep sense of grief that he was no longer physically a part of me. The kicks, the turns, the quiet companionship I'd grown so used to. My body, which had felt so full of life, now felt foreign and unfamiliar.

I looked down and didn't recognize what I saw: the bruising; the still-swollen tummy; the C-section scar stitched across soft, loose skin. The bump that had once brought smiles and glowing compliments was gone, and in its place was silence. Nobody cooed over this version of my body; nobody admired it anymore. In that moment, I was hit by the realization of how fleeting the celebration of the pregnant body really is, and how quickly it turns from something sacred to something scrutinized.

Over the course of the next two weeks, I rapidly lost all the water retention and was practically chained to the toilet – I couldn't stop weeing. Everyone around me told me how slim I looked; how I was the same size as I was before pregnancy and how remarkable that was. I remember the midwife telling me at the six-day post-birth check-up that she couldn't believe I had been pregnant because my stomach was so flat. But honestly? After the initial shock of confronting my new body, I couldn't have cared less about what people were saying about how I looked. Any thoughts of body image were well and truly buried under a truckload of hormones I had no control over, debilitating postpartum anxiety, and coming to terms with being wholly responsible for an entire human being. Who had signed that off?!

It was only a good few months later, when I began to feel more confident in looking after a baby, and more emotionally and mentally stable, that I realized how much weight I had gained *after* giving birth. Yep, that's right – not during pregnancy, but after. It's not something we hear about, is it? There's endless commentary and conversations around 'baby weight', but it's always assumed to be the weight gained *during* pregnancy – the kind of weight gain that's temporary and expected, to a certain extent. But after pregnancy, when everyone expects you to be 'bouncing back', it really goes against the grain to be getting bigger.

I felt like I'd been prepared for pregnancy weight gain and I'd made peace with it. But I wasn't prepared for postpartum weight gain. I thought it was just me this had happened to – that is, until I spoke about it on Instagram, received a huge response and realized it's incredibly common. It totally makes sense, of course: after giving birth, you're thrown into survival mode. You're adjusting to a completely new life, a new identity and a new level of pure exhaustion. For lots of us, we cope by turning to food for comfort, for a sense of control and a sense of relief.

I had never craved sugar so much as those few months after giving birth: I woke up dreaming of sugar and went to sleep thinking about it. Biscuits; chocolate; pastries: anything fast and sweet that gave me even a flicker of energy or pleasure in the haze of broken sleep, endless feeding and nap schedules. I wasn't eating with nutrition in mind or trying to fuel myself; I was eating to survive and to soothe – and I let myself, because it was what I needed at that time and that's OK.

We pathologize emotional eating, and I understand that binge eating can have a deeply detrimental effect on someone's life, but I truly believe that sometimes it's OK to use food for comfort, especially in seasons of life that are so physically and emotionally demanding, like the postpartum period. We're not robots; we don't live exclusively on perfectly-portioned protein bowls and green juices, and nor should we be expected to. Sometimes, what your body and mind needs is a cup of tea and a handful of biscuits at 8.00 a.m. when your baby *finally* goes down for a nap. I'd go so far as to argue that it's not failure, but self-care. After all, food *is* emotional. It's part of how we connect, socialise, celebrate, grieve, and cope. Of course, if food is your only coping mechanism, it's perhaps worth exploring and thinking about how you can expand your toolbox. But the idea that we can't somehow use food as one way to help get us through hard stretches feels unfair and disconnected from real life.

What makes all this so totally absurd is that the exact opposite is expected of us; that in the middle of this life-altering, exhausting, all-consuming transition into motherhood, we're also meant to . . . go on a *diet*? To restrict food, monitor calories, 'bounce back' and 'get our bodies back' – as if we've lost anything in the first place.

It wasn't just my weight gain that surprised me: it was the wider hips, the much larger boobs, and the softer stomach that looked completely different. My milk also never came in, and this realization that I wasn't going to be able to breastfeed my baby was a heartbreak I hadn't anticipated. Everyone around me was telling me that it didn't matter, and as long as he was fed, he was fine, but so much guilt and shame crept in anyway. Although the regimented idea of 'breast is best' is being challenged, there's a quiet cultural belief that breastfeeding is a measure of 'good' motherhood. When your body doesn't cooperate, it can honestly feel like failure. It's another standard that women are set up to internalize, and another way we're told our bodies should just 'work' the right way. If they don't, it's somehow on us.

All these changes to my body hit me hard – and I'm embarrassed to admit to that. *Shouldn't I be immune to body image pressure?*

My whole career revolves around challenging beauty standards, unpacking body image issues and helping people feel at peace in their skin. I've also had *years* of therapy since I was diagnosed with my eating disorder. I really thought I was past this. But motherhood, especially the earlier months, cracked me open in a way I wasn't prepared for. The physical changes were only part of it — they just happened to be the ones I could see.

In all honesty, I don't know if *anyone* is immune from it — not even those of us who have done, and continue to do, the work to address our relationships with our bodies. The culture we live in is relentless, and it doesn't discriminate. It doesn't skip over you just because you're aware of it — if anything, I think awareness can make it even harder at times, because you're battling both the feelings *and* the shame of having the feelings in the first place. The expectations placed on postpartum bodies are absurd — and yet, somehow, they're so embedded in our culture that we don't always realize we're internalizing them.

Nowhere is that more obvious than in the language we use — *bounce back*.

'Bouncing Back'

You've just done something that is really quite unbelievable — grown and delivered a whole human — and somehow, the world expects you to 'bounce back'. As if the most profound transformation your body can go through should leave no trace. You find the phrase everywhere. It's used so casually, like it's just part of the normal timeline of motherhood: baby groups, nappies, birth — bounce back. But our bodies are not rubber balls; they're not meant to *bounce.* They're meant to expand, adapt, heal and evolve. Pregnancy and birth rearranges your organs, shifts your bones, stretches your skin, alters your hormones and pushes you to your emotional, physical and often psychological limits. Why are we expected to look exactly the same afterwards? It's not just unrealistic, it's cruel.

Despite this, though, for so many women – particularly those in larger bodies – the pressure to restrict doesn't just come solely from societal or internal pressure, but from the medical system itself. Despite the vulnerability of the postpartum period, many women report being treated primarily for their size rather than their symptoms. Instead of receiving compassion or proper care, they're met with unsolicited weight-loss advice or lectures about BMI. Sometimes, it seems as though a woman's size is prioritized over her wellbeing. It's not always the fault of individual practitioners; many are operating within a weight-centric medical model, where BMI is treated as a shortcut for diagnosis and fatness is seen as a problem to be solved. But this approach causes harm at any life stage, and especially during postpartum, when what most women need most is nourishment, healing and mental health support.

Surely that should be the priority, not weight loss. We need to be asking mothers how they're coping emotionally, not how much weight they've lost.

I can't erase all physical signs of what happened to me – and I don't want to, either. Pregnancy is an experience that is forever integrated in my body. It's in my hips that widened to carry Tommy; in the skin that stretched to make room for him; and in the scar tracing across my stomach where he was lifted into the world. None of those are flaws; they're evidence of growth, of life and of survival. I want to honour them. And while I still have days where I long for the familiarity of my old body, what I've come to realize is that this new body has taken me through the best, most demanding and most transformative season of my life. It doesn't deserve criticism; it deserves respect and care and love.

And yet, we're bombarded with the 'bounce back' messaging at every turn, and the idea that, the quicker you can erase any signs of pregnancy or birth, the better. Your stomach should be flat; your face should be glowing with effortless 'mum life' vibes. The stretch marks? The soft belly? The wider hips? Airbrush them in photos. Hide them. *Fix* them.

Brands reinforce the pressure by marketing special 'mum-tum' shapewear, postpartum fitness guides and eating plans. Influencers will share 'before and after' video transformations, or reels of 'what I eat in a day' to 'get back to pre-pregnancy weight' – with captions that often include something along the lines of, 'no excuses, Mama!'. Even in NHS pamphlets, 'losing baby weight' is casually listed as a postpartum milestone alongside healing and bonding with your baby. Just the act of writing that makes me feel so sad. Then there's the quiet shame of being the only one in your NCT group not back in your pre-pregnancy jeans. There are the comments from family members who mean well but say things like, 'You'll bounce back in no time' or 'Once the baby weight is gone, you'll feel like yourself again'.

The Dad Bod

There's something deeply gendered in all of this. Enter: the 'dad bod.'

The dad bod is often defined as a man's physique that is fuller and softer, usually with a rounded stomach. It suggests a man who's not overly focused on fitness, who enjoys his food and doesn't obsess over calories or gym time. Far from being criticized, it's celebrated! The dad bod is framed as comforting, attractive and even aspirational – a surefire sign of a man who's confident and secure enough in himself, and so dedicated to his family that he doesn't have capacity to count calories or go to the gym. This man has his priorities straight: family, fun, and not worrying about abs. Pop culture embraces it, magazines joke about it, and partners are encouraged to find it sexy. There are no urgent headlines about 'snapping back' after becoming a dad; no diet plans marketed to help men erase the signs of parenthood; and no shame if the weight stays on, or if the body changes with time. If anything, it's a badge of honour.

Now compare that to the 'mum bod'. A mother's changing body is not interpreted as a sign of comfort or contentment; more often than not, it's viewed as a problem to be solved, a project to be worked on and something to apologize for and fix. The contrast is striking. One is admired for 'letting go' in the best way. The other is expected to hold on – tightly – to the unrealistic standards of youth and thinness.

Postpartum Bodies in the Media

Celebrity status certainly doesn't offer immunity from the scrutiny; in fact, the pressure is dialled up to an extreme when it comes to celebrity mothers. Postpartum bodies are treated like public property: dissected and turned into clickbait. A woman might be holding her newborn in one arm, but the headlines will be focused on her waistline. Articles about postpartum women are framed as progress reports: *Female celebrity* shows off post-baby body a week after giving birth' or 'She flaunts her incredible postpartum physique' – we see it again and again. While most of us will never face that level of public dissection, we still absorb the message. These stories trickle down and set the cultural tone for what's expected of *all* women after birth: to 'bounce back' and do it quickly.

Kate Middleton is another example. When she left the hospital after giving birth to Prince George in 2013, she was immediately scrutinized for her appearance. *OK! Magazine* ran a front-page story titled 'Kate's Post-Baby Weight Loss Regime', complete with a supposed 'Duchess diet' exclusive, revealing how her 'stomach will shrink straight back'. The implication was crystal clear: the clock is already ticking. The grace period of pregnancy is over, it's time to get back to work – not just as a royal, but as a woman who needs to reclaim her pre-baby body and 'look the part'.

And when women don't snap back – or just don't do it fast enough – the backlash comes just as swiftly. Take Hilary Duff. Just *three weeks* postpartum, she was photographed leaving Pilates and the internet tore into her for 'waddling'. It's worth mentioning here that, three weeks after giving birth to Tommy, I was so out of it, I honestly might as well have been on a different planet. Hilary didn't shrink back from the criticism, sharing a bikini photo to Instagram. Asked about it on the *Ellen* show, she said: 'I'm so proud of my body and what it's done for me. It gave me the most beautiful little boy, and I feel strong and powerful, and I wanted to inspire other women.'

It was genuinely refreshing to see someone in the public eye push back against the toxic bounce-back narrative with pride rather than defence. Hilary's words reframed the postpartum body as something to celebrate rather than fix and in an industry that rewards erasing the physical signs of motherhood, her openness felt necessary. She wasn't apologizing for looking different; she was reminding us that a body that's just grown and a birthed a human isn't a project to fix.

Sometimes, women don't even get to the postpartum stage before criticism hits. Margot Robbie announced her pregnancy in 2024, and when paparazzi pictures of her were published in a bikini, social media commenters were quick to cruelly judge her pregnant body. 'Margot Blobbie', one wrote. 'I feel so sorry for her husband', wrote another. Jessica Simpson is another example: during her pregnancies, the press *relentlessly* picked her apart for weight gain. Tabloids ran headlines calling her 'huge', 'bloated' and 'unrecognisable' and she became a punchline of late-night TV. Writing a blog post for *Parents.com* in 2013, Jessica wrote: 'My pregnancies (especially my first with Maxwell) were well documented and my struggles with my weight and body image have played out in front of the world.'

It was horrifying to watch, not just because of the cruelty she endured – I can't imagine how hard it must have been to be so openly mocked like that at such a vulnerable time – but because it sent a message to every woman watching it. It told us all that a woman's pregnancy is only acceptable if it is neat and photogenic. The reality of swollen ankles, stretch marks, puffy faces and extra weight was very, very explicitly treated as something shameful. For many of us who were pregnant or who hoped to be one day, watching that unfold felt like a warning.

And of course, we can't forget how Kim Kardashian was treated during her first pregnancy in 2013. The criticism was merciless: tabloids called her a 'whale' and claimed she'd be 'dumped' for being too fat, while social media users mocked her swollen feet and hands – which, it's worth adding, was due to pre-eclampsia, a serious pregnancy complication. Someone on Twitter (now X) even posted a photo of her wearing a black and white dress side by side with a picture of a whale: 'Who wore it better – Kim Kardashian or Shamu the whale?', read the caption.

Two years later, Kim opened up about the impact of that period on her self-confidence. 'It was the worst,' she told *C Magazine*. 'I couldn't help it, and everyone would say, "She can't stop eating"... they were like, "She's 210 pounds. She's getting dumped because she's too fat" and all these ridiculous stories. It really took a toll after the fact.'

Having built a career in harmony with the paparazzi, Kim suddenly found herself unable to engage with them. 'Before I was always smiling, and so into being out and about,' she said. 'After I had the baby, I was like, these are the same people that made fun of me, and posted the stories that were so awful, calling me fat for something I couldn't control. I don't want to smile for them. I don't want to be out. Even if I was more confident, I just didn't feel like that girl who was going to be smiling for every photo. It changed my mood; it changed who I was; it changed my personality a lot.'

Rihanna isn't immune from the criticism either. Just seven months after giving birth to her second child, she was branded 'lazy' after performing at a pre-wedding party in India, and there was rampant speculation that she was pregnant again because her stomach wasn't, well, completely flat. Let's take a second to think about that: she had recently grown and delivered a whole human, returned to the stage for her first full concert in nearly a decade, and the entire focus was on her body. She had either failed to 'bounce back' or she was pregnant again – because, apparently, those are the only two options when a woman's stomach isn't visibly concave.

This is all horrifying, but here's where, arguably, it gets worse: what happens when a woman *does* meet the ideal? When her body 'snaps back' in all the ways we've been conditioned to applaud? Well, of course, she gets criticized too.

Shortly after giving birth to her son, Emily Ratajkowski posted a photo of herself looking slim, essentially – and the internet exploded with fury. 'This is so unrealistic,' commenters wrote. 'You're making other mums feel bad.' 'Stop promoting toxic bounce-back culture.'

Now look, I understand where this frustration comes from – it *is* damaging to only ever see thin, flat-tummied postpartum bodies in the media and for that to be portrayed as the norm. But Ratajkowski wasn't promoting anything; she was simply sharing a photo of her body. The outrage revealed something complex, and frustrating: we punish women not just for failing to 'bounce back', but also for bouncing back too fast, or too visibly. Once again, it's a no-win game. A woman shows up postpartum in a body that hasn't 'bounced back' and she's shamed. A woman shows up postpartum in a body that has, and she's shamed again.

The Reality of Postpartum Recovery

What gets lost in all of this noise is the reality: postpartum recovery looks different for everyone. Genetics, birth experiences, mental health, support systems, access to childcare, class, race, privilege – all these factors, and more, play a role in postpartum recovery. Then there are the hormones. Wow, the hormones. I've never been so knocked off my feet by hormones as I was after giving birth.

To get a full picture of what happens to the hormones in the body around pregnancy and postpartum, I spoke to hormone and integrative medicine doctor, Sohère Roked. 'Pregnancy and postpartum is an incredible hormone rollercoaster,' she says. 'When you first become pregnant, you're flooded with oestrogen and progesterone and by the third trimester, oestradiol (oestrogen) can be up to 100 times higher than pre-pregnancy levels.'

But the levels don't just taper off gently: 'Within 24 hours after giving birth, these hormones plummet, which can cause baby blues, which is marked by tearfulness, irritability and fatigue, and some can even get postnatal depression if they're unable to regulate that hormone crash.' Studies show that 85 per cent of new mothers experience 'baby blues' while 10–20 per cent develop full postpartum depression. And that's not all we're dealing with. 'Cortisol and other stress-related hormones can then spike as is expected for a new mother as she attempts to navigate life with a brand-new baby,' explains Sohère.

We're still not done with the hormonal changes: 'If you're breastfeeding, your body will release more prolactin, the hormone which stimulates milk production – but it doesn't just affect your breasts. Prolactin can also suppress ovulation, reduce libido and contribute to feelings of fatigue or emotional flatness,' says Sohère. 'It can take a long time for your hormones to return to their normal cycle. For some women, it can take up to 18 months, and I often see mothers in clinic whose hormones have never returned to their baseline.'

These dramatic hormonal shifts are seismic, and they impact

mood, metabolism, appetite, sleep, healing, and emotional regulation. Your body and brain have just done something that resets your entire physiology, and yet, we demand that women simply . . . bounce back?

Postpartum Identity

The physical transformation of having a baby is only half the story. What is covered less is the identity shift – one that I wasn't prepared for at all. There's a strange kind of limbo after you give birth, where the world wants to celebrate you – but only as a mother. The person you used to be, with your own needs and goals? All this suddenly becomes irrelevant, because you are a *mother* now, and that shift in how you're perceived is so apparent.

Suddenly, everything is about the baby, and rightly so, in many ways – they're tiny, fragile and entirely dependent. But there's also this subtle erase of *yourself* that begins to creep in. People stop asking how you are, except in relation to how the baby's doing. Your entire being is absorbed into this new role – in a way that just doesn't happen for dads, sadly.

That imbalance shows up everywhere: mothers are expected to breastfeed, tend to the baby's every need and be endlessly nurturing and selfless, all while recovering physically and emotionally from birth. Fathers, meanwhile, often return to work after two short weeks, leaving the woman by herself. This isn't necessarily an active choice by fathers, but rather a byproduct of a culture that still positions men as the breadwinners and women as the carers.

As I write this, I'm nineteen months postpartum – I swore I

would never count in months, but honestly? I do a lot of things now that I swore I'd never do – and I'm still not entirely sure I have a full grasp on 'who' I am. Does that sound dramatic? Maybe. But having a baby cracks you wide open and leaves you alone to put all the pieces back together – and it's *hard*. Of course, you *do* have a new identity – you can't be the person you once were, it feels impossible. You have a brand-new role, one that's important, and often it's all-consuming. That can be hard to reconcile with the version of yourself that existed before – the one who had autonomy, spontaneity, a sense of freedom you didn't even realize you had, and honestly, the version of you who had a whole lot less to worry about.

It's worth saying here that I wouldn't trade it for the entire world. I love Tommy with all my heart and soul and beyond, and there is nothing on this earth that has the capacity to bring me such joy in the smallest, most mundane of ways. But there is something about becoming a mother that asks you to set aside a lot of yourself, and it often feels as if you're just kind of left to find your way back.

I think this is a good time to acknowledge a different experience that some of you might well have had with your postpartum body: one dominated by control. When you feel untethered from the identity you knew before, it's tempting to grasp for something tangible; something you can control. For a lot of women, that becomes their body size. Focusing on weight can feel like anchoring yourself to something familiar, and that urge is totally understandable, even without the bucketloads of societal pressure on postpartum women. We've been conditioned our entire lives to see weight as marker of success, worth and discipline, so in the chaos of new motherhood, when you feel lost, or invisible, or just out of control, it makes total sense that shrinking yourself can feel like gaining something back.

And of course, with weight loss comes compliments: 'You look amazing!', 'You've bounced straight back!'. All these are little hits of validation in a season of life that otherwise offers little external reward. You're not sleeping, you're overwhelmed, you're navigating a seismic shift in your identity – but at least you're thin. And if people are praising you for that, it must mean you're doing something right – right? But this version of control is deceptive. I'd argue that it's merely an illusion of control. What you're doing is trying to outrun the discomfort of change, and the truth is that your body was *never* the problem. Your disorientation, your unmet need for support or validation, your pure exhaustion – those are the things that need tending to, not the softness of your stomach or the width of your hips.

As I write all of this, I wonder, genuinely, how we even get through this time. How we carry all of it: the physical recovery, the emotional rawness, the relentless responsibility, the invisible labour, the identity shift, and still manage to show up, day after day, and keep a tiny human alive.

I'm also really conscious of not wanting to discourage women from having children, or to paint early motherhood as nothing but hardship, because that isn't true. There is so much joy – sometimes it's so intense that it almost knocks the breath out of you; the feelings of love and connection are so deep it can feel unbelievable. That said, I think we do women a disservice when we gloss over the harder bits; when we pretend that this transition doesn't also come with grief, or rage, or confusion.

Postpartum Intimacy and Sexuality

There's another layer to all of this – one that's rarely spoken about but felt – and often deeply. What does it mean to feel desirable again, and to explore sex and sexuality after giving birth?

The postpartum body is tender territory, to say the least. You're dealing with a body in recovery in so many different ways – healing pelvic floor muscles, stretched or separated abdominal muscles, C-section scars, perineal tears, leaking breasts, painful nipples and hormonal upheaval. Within all of this, there's often very little room left for pleasure, or sensuality, or even desire. Yet, at six weeks postpartum – just *six weeks* after your body has undergone perhaps the most physically intense experience it will ever go through – you're told you can have sex again! It's a strange medical green light that seems to ignore vital questions like, 'How are you feeling in your body?', or 'Do you feel ready yet?' If most women's postpartum experience is anything to go by, the answer is usually 'no': stitches and exhaustion aren't exactly conducive to physical intimacy.

Readiness isn't just physical, either. That medical green light isn't always accompanied by desire, and there are emotional complexities at play, too, that can make intimacy feel complicated. Maybe your partner doesn't know how to approach you anymore, or maybe you don't know how to receive it. 'The six-week check-up might confirm a physical readiness, but in no way does it indicate psychological readiness – and this is the biggest issue that should be named, validated and discussed with the couple,' says clinical psychosexologist Catriona Boffard. 'Many women are not ready – let alone able – to engage intimately with their partner at this time.'

In my experience, it's also so much easier to pull away from physical touch when your body feels unfamiliar. 'I'm yet to meet a woman whose views of her body have not changed postpartum,' says Catriona. 'While no two women are the same in how they experience their bodies, every body has been through a systemic change. How you feel about and in your body is directly linked to your ability to let in and let go when you are intimate. Touch can even feel completely different postpartum, and your needs may have changed. We cannot separate our bodies and brains, and both matter when we're getting physical with our partner.'

I asked Catriona what advice she has for women who don't feel at home in their bodies, let alone comfortable being intimate: 'Give yourself the same gentleness and kindness that you would give a friend,' she says. 'Your body has gone through immense change; it is normal not to feel comfortable. Be honest if you're battling and ask your partner for what you need, whether that's more patience, understanding or more compliments. Allow yourself to consider that your needs might be different now and that you need to adapt to meet yourself where you're at, rather than forcing yourself into anything because "everyone else does it so I should".'

Realistic Representations of Postpartum Bodies

There is just *so* much about pregnancy and postpartum that requires an open conversation that allows mothers to feel seen and supported. When it feels like our reality is missing from the cultural narrative, it's easy to feel like we're the only ones struggling.

It's not just the conversations that are missing, either – it's the images. Think about it: how often do you see an honest visual depiction of a body after birth? The leaking breasts, the scar tissue, the stretch marks and the swollen bellies; the adult nappies (and the weird floral smell of them?! That has stayed with me!), the hair loss, the hormonal acne – all of it. These bodies are everywhere in real life – but almost *nowhere* in media. We don't see accurate representations in films, in adverts, and barely even on social media accounts. There is a growing movement to show more honest postpartum content, and that's wonderful, but it's still not enough, especially not when it comes to bodies that are larger; bodies from different racial backgrounds; disabled bodies; or trans and non-binary bodies. These are the postpartum bodies we *never* see, and this kind of visibility really does matter – for validation, for reassurance; to know that our reality is represented and that it's *OK*.

Postpartum bodies also really deserve to be recognized – not hidden or airbrushed, not 'fixed' or transformed back into some version of their former selves; just seen, in all their glory. Because there is *so much* glory in these bodies – not in spite of what they've been through, but because of it. This brings me all the way back around to the cultural demands to 'bounce back', or 'get your body back' after giving birth.

What we're saying here, when we use these terms, is that our current body – the one that just performed a miracle – is somehow less valid than the one we had before. Let's be very, very clear: our body never went anywhere. It didn't vanish; rather, it grew, stretched, tore, and created and carried life. The idea that we need to revert to looking like we did before frames those changes as failures, rather than extraordinary feats. We've been taught to mourn our changed bodies, and whilst I do absolutely think there's space to grieve the past version of your body – I think that's healthy and a great step in moving forwards with your body image – to simply see the new version as a failure or a move away from worthiness is so damaging. What if the measure of postpartum 'success' wasn't how quickly we could shrink, but how deeply we could heal? What if recovery wasn't framed as returning to our old bodies, but instead focused on gently, patiently discovering who we've become?

'If we let go of the harmful idea that postpartum success means bouncing back to our old body, routine, energy or productivity, we open the door to a much more compassionate and truthful definition of success,' says Zoe Blaskey, a qualified transformational coach and speaker on modern motherhood. 'Instead, success could look like: learning to honour our needs without guilt, asking for help and receiving it without shame, allowing ourselves to rest, feel, grieve, celebrate – redefining our identity on our terms, not society's timelines and feeling connected to ourselves, our baby and our friends and family.'

Zoe adds: 'Motherhood is not something to "get through" (the definition of "bounce back" is to recover quickly from a setback: our babies aren't a setback) while trying to reclaim our pre-baby selves – it's a profound transformation. So, rather than bouncing back, what if we allowed mothers to move forward, slowly and supported, into a new version of themselves?'

What if we saw our new bodies not as failures but as evidence of creation, of survival and of endurance? The postpartum body tells a story. Every scar, every stretch march, every soft fold . . . it's a testament to life, and we deserve better than to be told to erase it or smooth it over or hide it under shapewear and layers of shame. We deserve a culture that doesn't *just* celebrate the bump, but honours what comes after, too. One that acknowledges the mother, yes, but also the woman *behind* the role. A culture that just doesn't focus on six weeks of aftercare and expect us to go forth and pretend that our bodies – and lives – haven't been entirely rearranged.

I'm not sure that there's a clear timeline to the postpartum period, honestly, because what we're really moving through is something called 'matrescence': the physical, emotional and psychological transition into motherhood. 'Some mothers find matrescence a much simpler process to navigate, while others can really struggle (depending on so many factors from child health to mental health to support levels) and it honestly can take years to feel confident and capable again,' says Zoe.

It's a process, the work of matrescence, and there's no one-size-fits-all path through it.

So, What Can We Do?

I think that we start by having open, candid conversations about postpartum. When we're struggling, I think it's vital that we can say out loud exactly how we're feeling and try to connect not only with those in our support networks but also with other new mothers who are having similar experiences. That connection is powerful and can end up being a lifeline for some.

We *have* to reject the bounce-back narrative – with our words, but also with our actions: by choosing clothes that fit well and that we feel comfortable in, rather than squeezing into old ones; by unfollowing social media accounts that make us feel bad; and by monitoring the way we talk to ourselves. A great rule of thumb to hold onto is that, if you wouldn't say it to someone you love, you don't deserve to say it to yourself either.

We need to start seeing our postpartum bodies not as a problem to solve, but as a powerful testament to what they achieved. They deserve compassion, love, respect and care and they are something to honour. We don't need to treat signs of life as flaws, like we've been taught.

If you're currently in the thick of it, mourning the body you had and struggling with the one you're in now, and all the while navigating a messy, emotional return to yourself, please know that it gets better and know too that you deserve so much compassion. It's great to seek it from others, but it's vital that you are the person who can give yourself that compassion unconditionally, too.

We don't need to bounce back. We don't need to 'get our bodies back'. They never went anywhere.

The Headlines
- Pregnancy and birth transform the body in profound and often permanent ways far beyond what we are ever prepared for
- The celebration of the pregnant body is fleeting while the scrutiny of the postpartum body is relentless and deeply unfair
- The pressure to 'bounce back' is rooted in misogyny, unrealistic beauty standards and a culture that treats women's bodies as projects rather than living, evolving organisms
- Postpartum weight gain, rather than weight loss, is common, normal and often driven by survival, hormones, exhaustion and emotional need – not a lack of discipline
- The hormonal upheaval after birth is seismic: mood, appetite, libido, sleep, metabolism and emotional regulation are all dramatically affected
- Postpartum identity is complex: alongside joy and heart-expanding love sits grief, disorientation and often a loss of sense of self that requires support and compassion
- Healing – physical, emotional and psychological – takes far longer than six weeks, and no two postpartum journeys look the same
- The postpartum body is not something to 'get back' from – it's living, breathing proof of creation, endurance and transformation, and it deserves to be honoured, not erased

A Moment of Reflection
- *What did I believe my postpartum body 'should' look like, and where did those beliefs come from?*
- *Did I feel more celebrated for my body pregnant than after giving birth? What did that shift feel like?*
- *What expectations did I place on myself because I thought they were 'normal', not because they were compassionate?*
- *Whose approval was I hoping to earn by 'bouncing back'? And do those values align with what I want for myself now?*
- *What would it look like to honour the body I have today, instead of mourning the body I had before?*
- *What would I want my child – or any future child – to learn by watching how I treat my own postpartum body?*

Where Do We Go From Here?

Postpartum is a really complex and messy period and we have to allow ourselves to feel all the complex and messy emotions without judgement or shame. It's OK to grieve our old bodies, and it's OK to miss who we were. But know that we can make choices that honour who we are now and offer ourselves the most compassion possible – at a time, quite frankly, where we couldn't need anything more.

We can choose clothes that fit the bodies we have now; we can unfollow accounts on social media that feed comparison; we can question the 'shoulds' we've absorbed and replace them with kindness and gentleness.

And, really importantly, we can begin to see postpartum not as a brief recovery period, but as a stage of matrescence: a long, layered, human process of becoming. There is no timeline, and no finish line. Just a slow becoming, shaped by love, exhaustion, new identity and unimaginable growth.

Your body didn't go anywhere. It carried life, delivered life, and continues to sustain your own. It deserves tenderness and it deserves patience, and it deserves reverence.

And you deserve all of that too.

Chapter 5

The 'Perfect' Face

We're entering a new era of beauty: one shaped by algorithms. This is the AI effect. Increasingly, the bodies and faces we compare ourselves to on social media and in adverts aren't even real. In today's beauty landscape, we're contending with representations of beauty that don't exist in human form, and ideals that are being generated by machines.

It's no secret that beauty has long been enhanced by technology. Early photography used chemicals and physical manipulation of negatives as retouching techniques, while the twentieth century saw the rise of soft-focus lenses and airbrushing during Hollywood's golden age, turning actors into impossibly smooth images of perfection. In the 1990s, Photoshop revolutionized image manipulation, allowing any flaw to be removed at the click of a mouse, and by the 2010s, Facetune and Instagram filters meant that those tools were no longer the reserve of models in magazines or celebrities – suddenly, they were in everyone's hands.

This evolution gave rise to what writer Jia Tolentino coined

The 'Perfect' Face

'Instagram Face' in a *New York Times* article, a hyper-specific, homogenised look that took over our feeds in the 2010s: skin that appeared impossibly flawless, heavy, arched brows, feline, almond-shaped eyes, long fluttery lashes, a button nose, high sculpted cheekbones, plump pillowy lips and a perfectly symmetrical face. This composite of features, many of them genetically rare, became the default aspiration and the epitome of beauty.

But the advent of AI has taken this phenomenon to an entirely new level and it's created beauty standards on steroids: while Instagram Face was the human version of perfection, painstakingly built through make-up, injectables, filters and Facetune, AI skips the human part entirely. It doesn't just enhance what's already there; it can construct beauty that was never even real in the first place. And there are no limits to what it can do.

Artificial intelligence has been positioned as beauty's next frontier. Industry press releases celebrate it as a revolution: personalized skincare routines tailored to your DNA; virtual assistants that help you find your 'perfect' lipstick shade; hair-care suggestions that respond to environmental changes – the list is endless. AI, we're told, will make beauty more efficient, more accessible, more *you*. But there's a darker edge too, one that isn't being shouted about quite so loudly. Because beneath the gloss of innovation lies a system that's quietly reinforcing the same old standards, only now, it does so more efficiently, more pervasively and under the reassuring guise of science and 'personalization'.

AI's influence on beauty didn't arrive overnight – it's been building quietly for years. What started out as early experiments in computer-generated modelling has steadily evolved into an industry – perhaps not a fully-fledged one just yet, but an industry nonetheless – that is creeping into every corner of our digital lives. AI-generated faces stare back at us from skincare ads and billboards; clothing brands use AI bodies to model outfits; and AI influencers sell us products from feeds that look indistinguishable from real-life content creators. The images are flawless and completely frictionless, devoid of the human realities of texture, pores, wrinkles, scars, stretch marks or even the subtle asymmetries that make real faces unique.

How Did We End Up Here?

The first real iteration of AI that hit the public domain was in 2016 with Lil Miquela, a freckled, fashionable 20-year-old influencer from Los Angeles, who quickly amassed a huge following on Instagram (she now has 2.4 million followers). She was thin, youthful and ethnically ambiguous with doll-like features and poreless texture. Miquela posed in Prada, attended music festivals, dropped singles on Spotify and hung out with celebrities like Bella Hadid. The twist? Lil Miquela wasn't a real person – she was a computer-generated character created by a Los Angeles start-up called Brud, designed to look, act and post like any other influencer, except every image was meticulously crafted on a screen.

Her success cracked the door open for other virtual influencers to enter the scene, including Shudu Gram, widely considered to be the world's first digital supermodel. Shudu was created in 2017 by British photographer Cameron-James Wilson, and she

The 'Perfect' Face

quickly gained a massive Instagram following, with many not even realizing she wasn't human. Within two years, Shudu had been featured in *Vogue* and *WWD*, fronted campaigns for Balmain and Ellese, and graced her first red carpet at the 2019 BAFTA film awards wearing a bespoke gown by Swarovski.

By 2019, AI- and 3D-generated influencers were no longer a novelty. Imma, a pink-bobbed Japanese virtual model created by Aww Inc., began fronting campaigns for IKEA, Puma and Valentino and even walking digital runways for Tokyo fashion brands. Her hyper-real skin texture, complete with freckles and the occasional blemish, blurred the line even further between reality and fabrication.

While these early digital women were unnerving, it's worth noting that they didn't always fit neatly into the mould of traditional beauty standards. Some, like Imma, had unconventional touches – a bold, pink bob haircut, freckles, visible skin texture – while Shudu was Black with deep, dark skin – in striking contrast to the overwhelmingly white, Eurocentric beauty ideals still dominating the fashion of the time. Yes, they were still products of an industry obsessed with visual perfection, but they carried hints of realism and, in some cases, intentional diversity. Perhaps it's telling that these supposedly 'progressive' figures were digital creations, rather than real women. In many cases, their creators were white men, which highlights an uncomfortable truth: inclusion was being simulated, not lived.

But in the years that followed, it seemed that AI moved away from these textured, diverse creations and started producing something more uniform: faces and bodies designed to embody a 'perfect' ideal.

Using AI in Our Everyday Lives

As AI evolved, so did the tools available to us as individuals. Filters used to be playful and fun additions to social media that felt harmless – a sprinkle of glitter or a silly dog face on a selfie. Today, AI-powered beauty filters go far beyond simple embellishment; they have the power to actively reshape our faces and our bodies. With one tap using AI, apps can slim your nose, lift your cheeks, sharpen your jawline, brighten your eyes, smooth your skin and whiten your teeth. A 2021 City University of London study found that 90 per cent of young women regularly use filters or photo-editing apps before posting.[14] We're no longer using filters to play, but rather to render ourselves 'perfect' beyond what is humanly possible, and to compete in an increasingly AI-generated world.

The consequences of our AI usage are stark. In research covered by NBC, 94 per cent of young women reported that filters caused pressure to look a certain way, with 75 per cent stating that they felt they 'would never live up' to those images, and 60 per cent reporting feelings of depression linked to filter use.[15]

What makes these statistics even more concerning is that recent research shows our brains are far less discerning than we might think when it comes to beauty, whether it's real or artificial. Studies using functional MRI scans have found that viewing attractive faces, whether real or digitally created, activates the brain's reward system, the same areas involved in pleasure, desire and reinforcement learning.[16] It turns out that we're not great at spotting the difference: one 2022 experiment found that participants could only correctly identify AI-generated faces about

The 'Perfect' Face

48 per cent of the time – essentially, no better than chance.[17] In other words, even when we know, on an intellectual level, that an image is artificial, our brains still process it as if it's real, releasing the same cocktail of dopamine and stress hormones that drive comparison and self-evaluation. This helps to explain why AI-generated 'perfect' faces can leave us feeling just as inadequate as we might feel when seeing a real, incredibly beautiful person. It doesn't matter that we know it's not real; our brains still wonder if we should try to look more like them.

AI and Brands

The commercial applications of AI beauty have exploded. Virtual try-ons allow you to experiment with lipstick shades, foundation tones, brow shapes and even entire hairstyles from your phone or laptop. In theory, this could be a good thing – such tools can reduce product waste, save time in-store and offer a personalized shopping experience. It's convenience on demand, and it works: brands that offer virtual try-ons average 64 per cent fewer returns compared to those that don't.[18]

By 2023, major e-commerce platforms like Zalando and Boohoo began quietly introducing AI-generated models to display clothing in multiple body types and skin tones. Deep Agency, a virtual modelling agency launched that same year, offered brands entire catalogues of AI-generated models, available on demand, for a fraction of the cost of hiring human talent. And here's where it gets complicated: in many ways, AI can be used for good. In retail, for instance, it can be used to showcase clothing on a wide range of body sizes, shapes and different skin tones. This is notoriously expensive and time-consuming for brands to do with human models: while hiring human models for a single campaign can cost brands tens of thousands of pounds, AI-generated models cost mere hundreds. For a global fashion retailer, this represents savings of millions annually.

It's a compelling financial incentive – one that hits home for me. I used to have a brand called Light LDN, with my business partner Sian, which ranged from sizes 6-30. We wanted to model the clothes on as many different body sizes and shapes as possible because diverse representation was the foundation of our ethos. In reality, it was incredibly difficult and cripplingly expensive: hiring multiple models for each product, booking extra studio time, producing more samples and creating so much imagery added huge costs and logistical difficulty to every collection we released.

In the end, it was one of the reasons we had to close Light LDN. Because of our commitment to representation and our emphasis on sustainability, our prices had to be higher, and as a small business, we simply couldn't compete with the rock-bottom prices of fast fashion giants. Had the AI tools available today existed back then, we could perhaps have at least explored them. They might have made it possible for us to keep our commitment to showing clothes on different bodies without the prohibitive costs and perhaps given us a fighting chance in an industry that rewards speed and scale over values.

That said, I'm not blind to the ethical concerns here. For models, fighting AI misuse is tricky. In both the UK and the US, most professional models are classed as independent contractors, which means they can't legally form a union. But the Model Alliance, led by former model Sara Ziff, has been speaking out about the need for stronger protections, especially when it comes to using a model's image without permission. As Sara has noted in interviews, when a person's image is central to their livelihood, reproducing or selling it without consent represents a serious rights violation.

As well as the threat of misuse of model's images, replacing human models with AI-generated ones inevitably means fewer paid opportunities for real people in an industry where jobs are already few and far between. It's a complicated trade-off: representation matters deeply, but so does the livelihoods of the people providing it. In theory, AI could help smaller, values-led brands showcase genuine diversity without prohibitive costs, but in reality, the technology is more likely to be used by big corporations to simulate diversity while cutting costs – with models being the ones to bear the brunt. However we progress in this space, I think it's imperative that the people behind the technology – and the brands using it – are genuinely committed to fairness and representation.

The Economics of AI

When we step back, it becomes clear that this isn't just about who gets to model the clothes or whose face appears in the campaign; it's about who holds the power and who reaps the financial rewards.

The real reason for AI's existence in the beauty space is because it's profitable. The commercial model that underpins almost all online beauty content depends on a simple equation: the more inadequate we feel, the more money we spend. Insecurity is one of the most reliable drivers of purchasing. When we see AI-crafted faces of perfection that highlight the 'flaws' in our own, we're nudged towards products, procedures and services that promise to make us look more like them.

As with retail, the financial incentives for beauty are huge. Advertisers can now generate endless streams of homogenised beauty imagery at a fraction of the cost of working with real models, and at a scale no human workforce could match. This efficiency comes at a hidden cost, however: when algorithms optimize for speed and volume, they gravitate toward whatever patterns appear most frequently in their training data. And here's the catch: like all AI tools, their outcomes are only as inclusive as the data they're trained on – and the data sets aren't neutral. They're scraped from an internet already saturated with images that platform whiteness, thinness, youth and Eurocentric features, reflecting decades of advertising, fashion photography and influencer content that overwhelmingly centres on a very narrow ideal. So, it's no surprise that personalized beauty tools, which should reflect the full diversity of human faces, often converge on the same one. AI's tendency to produce a singular aesthetic: youthful, symmetrical, light-skinned, slim, smooth and vaguely ethnically ambiguous, is a composite face created from a formula born of repetition and bias. Then there's the matter of who's building these tools. The tech industry is still dominated by white, male engineers, and even when bias isn't intentional, it is unconsciously coded into the algorithms, which then churn out content reinforcing the very same ideals. We are presented with the illusion of choice, when in reality we're just being handed variations of the same digital doll.

AI in the Media

In 2025, *Vogue* sparked controversy with its August issue, which featured an AI-generated model in a Guess ad. The model was white, but had tanned, flawless skin, perfectly bouncy blonde hair, ultra-smooth, symmetrical features and a Hollywood smile. She epitomised everything I've ever wanted to look like and was the digital embodiment of everything we've been sold as the ultimate ideal. Social media lit up with criticism, calling out both the ad and the publication for recycling the same narrow beauty archetype we've been fed for decades, now dressed up in the glossy, pixellated packaging of AI.

The same bias was on full display at the first-ever Miss AI beauty pageant in 2024, which drew hundreds of AI-generated contestants from around the world. Despite being billed as a celebration of creativity and innovation, the finalists all looked eerily similar: perfectly symmetrical features, poreless skin, high cheekbones, plump lips, small noses. Most had slim bodies, long hair and Eurocentric features. Even those presented as 'diverse' were simply variations on the same digital template. Not one of the contestants displayed any kind of real body diversity, and even one of the judges, Sally-Ann Fawcett, a pageant historian, admitted that the line-up was lacking in representation: 'I would like to see somebody of a different gender, somebody larger, somebody older, somebody with flaws,' she told *NPR*.

In 2024, an ad campaign by Dove made AI's bias towards 'perfection' impossible to ignore. Designed to test beauty image generators, *The Real State of Beauty* experiment asked AI to create 'the most beautiful woman in the world'. The results? Across different prompts, locations and generators, the AI produced dozens of virtually indistinguishable women: young, thin, and white, with blonde hair, blue eyes, unnaturally flawless skin and immaculate symmetry. The Dove team analysed the AI outputs and found that only one in five images showed any visible skin texture.

These avatars also looked uncannily similar to the Guess AI model, providing further evidence that when beauty is filtered through machine learning, it doesn't expand our imagination; it narrows it. This is underscored by Dove's research, which reveals that 85 per cent of women already feel that AI beauty content is setting unrealistic standards, with 60 per cent saying they feel pressure to look a certain way because of what they see online.

AI and Diversity

These impacts aren't felt equally across all communities. Research shows that people of colour face additional pressure as AI beauty filters often struggle to accurately render darker skin tones, frequently lightening them or failing to work entirely. Meanwhile, the disabled community finds themselves almost entirely erased from AI beauty standards: when was the last time you saw an AI-generated face with a visible difference, a hearing aid, or any marker of disability?

This erasure is algorithmic. AI systems learn from datasets that reflect decades of exclusion in media and advertising. If the training data predominantly features young, white, able-bodied people, that's what the AI will replicate and amplify. For marginalized communities already fighting for representation, AI beauty tools can feel like another door closing.

Meanwhile, emerging research shows beauty filters are far from neutral. A 2024 study titled 'Mirror, Mirror on the Wall, Who Is the Whitest of All?' found that popular AI beauty filters tend to lighten skin and alter facial features in ways that prioritize white beauty standards, regardless of a user's cultural background.[19] This is particularly visible in markets like China, where filters have helped popularise a homogenised aesthetic comprising smooth skin, enlarged eyes and slim chins. The authors describe this phenomenon as a form of 'digital colonialism': the systematic imposition of Western beauty ideals through technology. They note that this 'Western-driven process presents the Western world as attractive and beneficial, while appropriating, homogenising, and standardising the Global South'. These algorithmic preferences echo the real-world legacy of racism – harmful skin-whitening creams and bleaching products (some still laced with mercury or steroids) remain widely marketed and sold across Asia, Africa and Latin America. It's striking how the tools may have changed, but the underlying message being sold is that lighter is still better.

Other studies from Ghana, Sri Lanka, and broader Asian contexts show that beauty filters and AI tools are amplifying Westernized beauty norms at the expense of local aesthetics. For instance, in Sri Lanka, AI filters reinforce historical preferences for lighter skin tones and reshape cultural beauty perceptions.[20] In Ghana, university students report frequent filter use driven by appearance ideals aligned with broader digital beauty trends.[21] Scholarship on the Westernization of beauty in Asia highlights how Western norms continue to dominate aesthetic standards across the region.[22]

Pressures to conform to Western beauty ideals are, of course, nothing new: colonialism, globalisation and Hollywood all exported narrow standards of 'attractiveness' *long* before AI existed, but what's changing is the mechanism of their enforcement. AI learns these ideals, replicates them and feeds them back to us at scale with algorithmic acceleration, reinforcing Western beauty as the default aesthetic setting. The idea that technology – something which could very well be a vehicle for celebrating and highlighting difference – is instead teaching us that beauty only exists within an exceptionally narrow framework, is incredibly unsettling.

We've seen before that meaningful representation is possible. For decades, mainstream beauty brands catered almost exclusively to white consumers, offering limited shade ranges that excluded huge swathes of women. When Fenty Beauty launched in 2017 with forty foundation shades, it sparked an industry-wide reckoning that should have happened decades earlier. Prior to this, MAC had made strides with a far wider shade range than most, but it was Fenty's success that showed the power of centring all skin tones rather than treating inclusion as an afterthought. The fact that AI threatens to reverse that progress is particularly jarring and concerning.

The Impact of AI in Beauty

One of the most insidious elements of AI in beauty is the fact that these tools purport to be objective. For instance, when an AI generator offers up your personal perfect lipstick match, or identifies the haircut that would best suit your face shape, it frames the output as a definitive, scientific fact, as opposed to a culturally influenced opinion. When a digital tool 'corrects' your skin tone, it frames the change as an improvement, rather than an aesthetic preference. AI has an authoritative framing that we trust. The consequence is that we internalize its suggestions, whether we buy the lipstick or not, and ultimately it can shape not only how we see others but how we see ourselves, because over time those micro-adjustments teach us that our unfiltered selves are the 'before' picture.

AI-generated beauty is also having a profound impact on how we feel. With an increasing proliferation of artificial representations that encompass the 'perfect' ideals of beauty, it doesn't matter if we know it's not real; our brain registers it and our body still responds to it. We still measure ourselves against it and compare ourselves to it, even if we don't mean to. This is the mental cost of perfection – dissatisfaction and detachment. There is an ever-widening gap between the body we live in and the one we present online; between who we really are, and who we're told we could be – if only we worked a little harder, spent a little more money, filtered a little more . . . It's exhausting.

Some experts warn that by 2030, all online content could be AI-generated, meaning that this narrowing of beauty ideals could quickly become inescapable. If these systems keep drawing from the same narrow pool of 'acceptable' features, the images we encounter every day will only grow more homogenised, more unrealistic and more detached from human reality.

The irony is that AI has the potential to make beauty more inclusive than it's ever been – to show us what clothes and products look like on every skin tone, every age, every body type – but without careful oversight and diverse data sets, it's far more likely to reinforce the narrowest ideals. The result? Billions of images that appear personalized but instead push everyone towards the same homogenous face and body and generate impossible ideals.

Throughout this book, we've covered the wealth of pressures that women are facing, and the toxic messages we receive from the outside world have remained remarkably consistent in their theme: your body and your appearance, as it naturally exists, is not enough. But AI beauty is uniquely troubling when compared with all the other pressures we've explored. Where previous beauty standards were at least theoretically achievable – you could, with enough money and surgery and discipline, potentially look like a celebrity or Instagram influencer – AI beauty offers us a vision of perfection that has never existed in human form. We're no longer competing with and comparing ourselves to enhanced versions of real people; now, the beauty standards we're facing are borne out of mathematical ideals generated by machines.

This feels like a culmination of generations of societal pressure; the logical endpoint of a culture that has spent decades teaching women that their value lies in their appearance. We've progressed from comparing ourselves to retouched magazine photos to filtered social media posts to entirely synthetic faces. Each step has moved us further from reality, and further away from the possibility of finding satisfaction, acceptance and peace with our own bodies.

I wonder how this is going to translate into our real lives? The data suggests that it's already resulting in more surgery, more tweakments, and more money spent chasing an impossible ideal, and inevitably, it is disproportionately impacting women. While men are increasingly seeking cosmetic procedures, women remain the primary target – and victims – of AI beauty standards. Across nearly every measure, research finds significant gender disparities in the use of beauty filters and editing tools, with women engaging more often and for longer durations than men.[23] This greater exposure comes at a cost: women report sharper increases in body dissatisfaction after viewing filtered or idealized images,[24] are more likely to compare their appearance to others on social media,[25] and show higher rates of self-objectification linked to frequent filter use.[26] In some cases, these pressures translate into tangible actions: studies show that women who regularly engage with image-based platforms like Instagram and Snapchat are more likely to express interest in, or undergo, cosmetic procedures, often inspired by filtered images of themselves.[27] The phenomenon of 'Snapchat dysmorphia' has become increasingly documented by medical professionals: Dr Neelam Vashi of Boston Medical Center coined this term to describe patients seeking cosmetic surgery to look like filtered versions of themselves. According to the American Academy of Facial Plastic and Reconstructive Surgery (AAFPRS), 55 per cent of surgeons report seeing patients who want to look better in selfies – up from 42 per cent just three years earlier. In short, the AI-accelerated beauty landscape doesn't just amplify existing inequalities, it deepens them.

For decades, women have faced exponentially more pressure around appearance than men, and AI is supercharging that inequality. While a man might use a filter to smooth his skin or whiten his teeth, women are increasingly feeling pressure to transform everything – their face shape, body proportions, skin tone, even their bone structure. The AI beauty tools reflect and amplify this disparity, offering women dozens of ways to alter their appearance while men's options remain relatively limited.

The economic implications of all this are staggering. Women already spend significantly more on beauty products, cosmetic procedures, and appearance-related healthcare than men. If AI beauty standards drive even more surgical interventions and beauty spending, it could create an even wider gender gap in discretionary income and financial security. We're potentially looking at a future where women feel compelled to spend ever-increasing amounts of money to compete with digital perfection – money that could otherwise go toward education, investments, or financial independence.

Perhaps the most urgent question isn't how this affects those of us who remember a pre-AI world, but what it means for the generation growing up within it. Children born today will never know a time when the majority of faces they see online were entirely human. They're developing their sense of beauty and their understanding of 'normal' in a world where digital perfection is becoming the baseline – it's an unprecedented time in human history and never before have beauty standards been so detached from reality.

Recent research reveals concerning trends among young people's relationships with digital beauty standards. A 2023 study published in *Frontiers in Psychology*, comprising 209 young people aged 16-18, found that image-based social media platforms were significantly associated with increased body dysmorphic symptoms.[28]

According to a 2023 study by Dove and the Centre for Appearance Research, 9 in 10 girls say they're exposed to beauty filters by age 13, and over half say they struggle to feel confident in their unfiltered appearance. Another study found that girls who regularly view filtered images are more likely to internalize unattainable beauty ideals and report increased anxiety, depression and self-objectification.

How Do We Move Forward?

The data may be bleak, but there is hope. This generation also has something we didn't: the potential to grow up with digital literacy. They can learn to recognize AI-generated content; be versed in the fact that algorithms have inherent biases and therefore aren't neutral. Perhaps they will be able to develop some immunity to digital manipulation because they'll understand it from the start. For that to happen, though, this awareness needs to be taught, and it's vital that education goes beyond simply telling young people, 'Don't believe everything you see online'. We need to see curriculums that teach media literacy, including AI awareness, and those of us with kids and young people in our lives need to include conversations about digital manipulation alongside more traditional talks about puberty, sex, and so on. The younger generations need to understand the economics of engagement, the history of beauty standards, and how that all feeds into digital manipulation.

We're already seeing resistance to AI: some brands are beginning to address public unease around AI's role in shaping beauty standards, and Dove became the first beauty brand to commit to never using AI-generated imagery to represent real people in its advertising. 'At Dove, we seek a future in which women get to decide and declare what real beauty looks like – not algorithms,' said Alessandro Manfredi, Dove's Chief Marketing Officer. 'As we navigate the opportunities and challenges that come with new and emerging technology, we remain committed to protect, celebrate, and champion Real Beauty. Pledging to never use AI in our communications is just one step. We will not stop until beauty is a source of happiness, not anxiety, for every woman and girl.'

Researchers are also working on improved methods for detecting AI-generated imagery. Digital forensic experts have spotted subtle clues – eye placement that feels slightly off, unnatural lighting or skin that looks too perfect – that give away computer-created faces. Social media companies like Meta say they're working on new detection tools, though they've shared little detail about how human reviewers are trained to spot the fakes.

Campaigners are calling for the introduction of increased rules and fairness around AI. The Algorithmic Justice League, set up by researcher Joy Buolamwini, works to make AI systems more transparent and less biased. In her *Gender Shades* study, Joy highlighted the biases within popular facial recognition software created by IBM, Microsoft and Face++. Her findings showed that, while the systems had a relatively high accuracy rate, there were vast discrepancies depending on skin colour and gender – that is, an error rate of just 0.8 per cent for white men, rising to 34.7 per cent for dark-skinned Black women,[29] proving these systems are far from neutral.

Change is also coming from the ground up. Digital literacy programmes are emerging that teach people how to recognize AI-generated content. Apps and browser extensions are being developed to help users identify when images have been artificially created or enhanced. Some platforms are experimenting with 'reality checks' – prompts that remind users when they're viewing heavily filtered or AI-generated content.

I'll be honest: researching and writing this chapter changed how I see every image I encounter online. I now find myself scrutinizing faces in advertisements, wondering if that model's impossibly smooth skin is the result of good genetics, professional retouching, or algorithmic generation. I catch myself questioning whether the influencer whose confidence I admire is even real, or whether I'm being sold an AI-generated fantasy. This constant vigilance may sound exhausting, but in this day and age, it's liberating. Once you understand how these systems work; once you see the bias baked into the algorithms and the commercial incentives driving the technology, you can't unsee it – and that awareness becomes a kind of armour.

I'm not saying I'm immune to the pull of digital perfection – I'm definitely not. I still sometimes find myself wishing I could use a filter before posting a photo, and there are inevitably those days where I catch my reflection and wish my skin looked as smooth as some of the faces in my feed. The difference is that I can now recognize these moments for what they are: the successful operation of systems designed to make me feel inadequate. I truly believe that this is where we find our power. Not in perfectly resisting every algorithmic manipulation, because, honestly, it's probably impossible in our hyperconnected world, but in developing a kind of digital discernment: the ability to pause, question, and choose our responses rather than react automatically to whatever impossible standard we're being shown.

The key is awareness. When we understand that the 'perfect' face staring back at us from our screens is often an algorithmic composite designed to sell us something, we can begin to resist its pull. When we know that the beauty filter 'recommending' a lighter skin tone or smaller nose is reflecting centuries of harmful bias rather than objective 'improvement', we can choose differently.

And when an AI beauty tool suggests 'improving' your appearance, you can stop and ask: *improve according to whom?* When a filtered selfie makes you feel inadequate about your own appearance, you can remind yourself: that's not what humans actually look like. When you find yourself poised to spend money on products or procedures to match a digital ideal, you can pause to question: *am I doing this for me, or for an algorithm?*

I don't believe we should reject technology entirely. AI beauty tools, designed ethically and with diverse input, could genuinely democratise beauty and representation, but we're not there yet. The key, therefore, is to demand better: to demand tools that celebrate rather than homogenise human diversity, to demand transparency about when and how AI is being used, and to demand that the future of beauty includes all of us, not just an algorithmic average.

The future of beauty doesn't have to be decided by Silicon Valley engineers and profit-driven algorithms. It can be decided by us – by our choices about what we'll accept, what we'll pay for, what we'll aspire to, what we'll fight against – but only if we stay awake to what's happening and refuse to let machines define our worth.

The 'Perfect' Face

The Headlines
- AI has entered the beauty space and threatens to completely redefine it, creating a new standard of 'perfection' that humans simply can't achieve
- Today's 'ideal face' is increasingly an algorithmic composite, shaped by biased datasets and built to maximize engagement
- AI-generated beauty erases texture, age, asymmetry and difference, often reinforcing Eurocentric, young, slim, light-skinned aesthetics
- Beauty filters and AI tools disproportionately impact women and girls, who experience sharper rises in body dissatisfaction, comparison and pressure to 'fix' themselves
- AI's commercial incentives are clear: the more inadequate we feel, the more money we spend
- Without ethical oversight and diverse data sets, AI risks reversing decades of progress in representation, inclusivity and self-acceptance

A Moment of Reflection

- *When I scroll through my feed, am I aware of the fact that I may be comparing myself to faces that aren't even human?*
- *What features do I find myself wishing for, and would I even desire them if algorithms didn't keep showing them to me?*
- *What does it do to my sense of self when my unfiltered face feels like the 'before' picture?*

Where Do We Go from Here?

We have to push ourselves to choose reality over 'perfection', even when perfection is so tempting. We can teach ourselves – and the next generation – to recognize AI, to build media literacy and to understand the economics behind the ideal. We can also demand better from the companies shaping our digital world, calling for diverse training data, transparency and tools that expand beauty rather than narrow it.

Most importantly, we can reclaim our right to look like humans: textured, asymmetrical, ageing, expressive, flawed, unique . . . We can embrace the joy in diversity and real, human, non-AI beauty in all its glory.

The future of beauty does not need to be defined by machines. It can be shaped by us: by our awareness, our boundaries, our choices and our refusal to let an algorithm decide our worth.

Chapter 6

Make-Up

In a world increasingly saturated with 'perfect', AI-generated faces, it's easy to blame technology alone for the pressure we feel to look a certain way. But these ideals don't *only* exist on our screens – they show up in our real lives too, and on our real faces, through the daily rituals we perform in the mirror. Make-up is arguably the original beauty technology, and even without AI, many of us – and overwhelmingly women – are still reshaping ourselves and altering our appearances, with the help of concealer, contouring, blusher, highlighter, lip liner.

Make-up has long been dismissed as frivolous; something surface-level, and a distraction from more serious things. It's been called vain, shallow, and unfeminist. Is make-up self-expression? A survival tool? Or simply conformity disguised as choice?

For many of us, make-up feels like freedom. It's fun and it's creative and it's a tool for self-expression. It can be part of a ritual, it can offer us joy, or even a form of therapy. The act of applying it can feel grounding – for many, it can feel like a way of taking control of your day or your mood. There's power in that, especially in a world that often tells women, trans people and marginalized genders *how* they should look, but rarely asks how they *want* to look.

I'd love to say that I fell in love with make-up precisely because of this creative potential, but I have to be honest and admit that the initial allure of make-up for me was grounded in its ability to make me look 'prettier', which at the time really meant 'more acceptable'. I reached for eyeliner, mascara and concealer not to explore artistry, but to hide my true features.

Make-Up and Me

My relationship with make-up began the same way so many young girls' and women's relationships do, as a means of survival in a world that constantly evaluates us visually. Make-up was the difference between feeling like I might pass unnoticed, or fearing I'd be judged for blemishes, dark circles or an uneven skin tone. I'm pretty sure that what I was really chasing was a sense of safety in conformity.

Somewhere along the way, though, that changed. I became a beauty editor for a magazine almost by accident. I'd been working as a fashion editor when an opportunity came up to cover the beauty desk, and I said yes. Suddenly, I found myself immersed in this new world. I started attending product launches, meeting make-up artists and watching them at work, testing new products before they hit the shelves and interviewing beauty experts from all corners of the industry. And I fell in love with it: I was genuinely excited by new innovations, curious about textures and formulas and fascinated by the science and the stories behind the products.

I stopped seeing make-up as a mask, and more as an exciting tool for creativity; somewhere technology and self-expression could converge in joyful and fun ways.

It didn't take long for another truth to sink in, though: behind the dazzling campaigns and empowering taglines, the people at the top of almost every major beauty corporation were middle-aged white men. And they weren't in the boardroom debating the nuances of self-expression or the cultural meaning of contouring; they were looking at profit margins. Inevitably, that profit came, overwhelmingly, from selling women the idea that we needed to look a certain way. My newfound love of beauty was real, but so was my growing awareness that this joy existed inside a system designed to monetise our insecurities.

That's the paradox at the heart of this topic: the very same products that can feel liberating and playful can also be the ones we reach for under pressure or fear of judgement. The lipstick that makes us feel bold on a Friday night might be the same one we feel obliged to wear to a Monday morning meeting because 'I look tired without it'. The same winged liner that feels like fun self-expression on a night out might feel like a mask on the morning school run.

This duality doesn't render make-up good or bad, but it does make it complicated. It also forces us to ask uncomfortable questions: *when I paint my face, is it because I want to, or because I've been taught that my bare face is incomplete? Am I adding something, or am I covering something up? Is this me, or is this me edited for public consumption?*

When you zoom out further, those personal questions become political ones. The fact that so many of us feel 'incomplete' without make-up isn't accidental; it's the outcome of a century of advertising, media, and now algorithms, all designed to keep us buying.

Surveys shows that 84 per cent of women report wearing make-up at least occasionally, and nearly half say they feel more confident when they do.[30] Psychology and sociology research point to several overlapping reasons why people reach for it, and they're rarely simple or singular. Some are personal, some are social.

On one end, there's the evolutionary argument: humans have always enhanced their faces to signal health, fertility and social status. But to leave the explanation there would be to ignore culture's say in deciding which features are celebrated and which are concealed.

For some, make-up is armour: a way to feel less visible to criticism, bias or even danger. A 2022 survey found that 45 per cent of trans women wear make-up most days, with many citing safety and gender affirmation as key reasons.[31] A jobseeker might apply concealer not to 'feel cute' but to avoid assumptions about tiredness or capacity – perceptions that research shows still disproportionately affect women in professional settings.[32] A teenager might do her eyeliner because, without it, she risks being called 'plain' in school.

For others, make-up is joy, self-expression, play and creativity. A non-binary person might use glitter and neon shadow to actively reject gender norms. A disabled woman might choose bright lipstick as a way of expressing her personality or sexuality in spaces where her body is otherwise hyper-medicalized. Many of us, regardless of background, find genuine pleasure in the textures, colours, packaging and the daily transformations that have nothing to do with anyone else's gaze.

Most of the time, I think our reasons sit in the overlap. Perhaps we start out wearing mascara to feel more acceptable and later find we love the drama of it. We might put on a lipstick for a night out because it feels fun, and also because we know it will be read as 'put together' in photos. I'm not sure that make-up is ever purely self-expression or self-protection. For most of us, it's both.

That doesn't mean there isn't a tension between the way make-up makes us feel and the reasons it makes us feel that way. Like so many things about beauty, identity and womanhood, it's layered, complex and often contradictory.

That messy intersection is most definitely where I land. I genuinely really *adore* make-up. Having an hour to myself to do a full face of make-up is a luxury (one that I rarely get time for now I have a child, but still!) and one that I treasure. I love trying out a new creamy blush, or the click of a heavy lipstick lid, and there is undoubtedly joy in the transformation that happens in the mirror. Well-applied make-up feels like art, and it's one of the very few rituals in my life that allows me that kind of creativity. I also have to admit that I almost never leave the house without it. Not because I think I'm too hideous without it, but because being seen bare-faced feels exposing and makes me feel incomplete.

The Politics of Make-Up

This is where the complex knot of make-up tightens – because I consider myself a feminist. I believe in dismantling beauty standards that restrict women's freedom, yet I still feel compelled to meet them most days. I write critically about the beauty industry, yet I've built parts of my career in partnership with it. I work with brands that I genuinely love – yet I know that some of those same brands profit from the insecurities that their marketing often helps to create.

So, how do I reconcile all of this? Can make-up ever truly be an act of feminism, or am I dressing up compliance as choice? Is it possible to still fight the system that tells me I need it? This is the question that has split feminist thought for decades.

Some still see make-up as a symptom of patriarchal control: a daily ritual of self-correction that keeps women's time, money and attention fixed on our appearance instead of our power. As Naomi Wolf wrote in *The Beauty Myth* (1990): 'Cosmetics are not a "luxury" as women are told, but an economic necessity to compete for work, status and security.'

Feminist scholar Sandra Bartky, meanwhile, argued that beauty work – including make-up – is one of the 'disciplinary practices' that keep women focused on self-surveillance, subtly enforcing compliance with patriarchal ideals.

Under this view, the £336 billion global beauty industry cannot be considered harmless fun; rather, it's a powerful economic system built on conditioning women to doubt their worth without a painted face. The statistics somewhat support this: research shows that women who wear make-up are often perceived as more competent, more likeable and more hireable in professional settings, making make-up a form of social currency.

But that's not the whole story. Many feminists – and many women – argue that make-up can also be a tool of self-definition and pleasure. As writer and feminist Chimamanda Ngozi Adichie has said, 'If she likes make-up, let her wear it . . . Don't think that raising her feminist means forcing her to reject femininity.'

And writer Roxane Gay: 'I wear lipstick because I want to. Because it makes me feel good. That's enough.' Feminist poet Audre Lorde framed self-care as 'an act of political warfare', and for lots of people that extends to beauty. A red lipstick, a winged liner or an iridescent swipe of highlighter can be an assertion of self in a world that tries to define you before you've even opened your mouth.

Make-up is not, and has never been, just a cis woman's issue. Trans and non-binary people have long used cosmetics to affirm their gender identity, to claim space in a society that increasingly polices gender presentation, and as something to protect themselves from violence.

Ultimately, it seems clear that the meaning of make-up is never fixed. The intent, the context and the personal history we bring to make-up changes everything.

This is why I think the 'is make-up feminist?' debate can never be answered with a simple yes or no. The reality is far more complicated and nuanced. Make-up exists within a patriarchal system, yes – but it can also be a way to subvert that system, to play with identity or to simply bring yourself joy on an otherwise grey and gloomy Tuesday morning.

Perhaps the more interesting question isn't whether make-up is feminist, but whether we are free to truly choose it. Would I still reach for my concealer every day if I had never learned that dark circles were undesirable? Would I still paint my lashes with mascara every morning if I hadn't learned that long, thick and fluttery lashes *were* desirable?

Make-up can be a way of pushing back, of claiming space and of presenting yourself to the world in a way that feels truest to you – whether that's with rainbow eyeshadow and glitter brows or just the tiniest bit of concealer over a particularly stubborn spot. But here's the catch: even our most joyful expressions are shaped by invisible pressures.

We don't always arrive at our preferences in a vacuum; we've been absorbing messages about what's 'beautiful', 'polished', 'presentable' and 'professional' since we were old enough to idolize Disney princesses or flip through a teen magazine. So, when we say, 'I wear make-up for me', we have to take a second to ask: who taught us what 'looking like me' should mean?

The Performance of Beauty

There's a fine line between expressing who you are and performing who you think you're supposed to be. Think about how we rarely see barefaced women in the media – unless it's as a 'before' photo, right? Think about how often a 'no make-up' look still involves at least ten different products. Or how compliments like 'you look fresh' or 'you're glowing' often translate to: you've successfully enhanced your face without appearing to try too hard.

So even when it feels like we're choosing, many of us are choosing from a very narrow selection. And more often than not, that selection leads us to the same place: smooth skin, long lashes, contoured cheekbones, plump lips, tamed brows. A more symmetrical, less tired, more sculpted, more 'acceptable' version of ourselves.

And there's nothing wrong with that – until it becomes the only version that we feel safe showing to the world.

The frenzied noise around Pamela Anderson in recent years is a perfect example of how loaded the conversation around make-up is. When she started to attend red carpets and magazine covers barefaced, it made headlines worldwide – she was applauded by some as brave and authentic, and criticized by others who saw it as a publicity stunt. The intensity of the reaction revealed how unusual it still is for women – especially women who built careers on beauty – to be seen without make-up in public. The fact that it became newsworthy says everything about the expectations we live under – a woman in the public eye being seen without make-up is so rare that it feels like a radical act of rebellion.

While Pamela Anderson may be on the front row at Paris Fashion Week or on the red carpet at the SAG Awards, the dynamic she exposes isn't reserved for celebrities. Her bare face became international news, but ours might draw a raised eyebrow from a colleague who asks, 'are you OK?', or a 'you look tired' comment from a friend, or a general sense that we're somehow presenting ourselves as being less polished or less professional. The stakes are different, sure, but the pressure is the same: our bare faces still read as incomplete.

And this isn't just about a personal choice; it's a billion-dollar tension that entire industries are invested in keeping unresolved. The cosmetics market was estimated at approximately $336 billion in 2024 and is projected to grow to over $556 billion by 2032.[33] Make-up accounts for a substantial slice of that total, feeding a sector dominated by a handful of multinational conglomerates: companies like L'Oréal, Estée Lauder, Procter & Gamble, and Unilever.

In the USA, the spending is significant. One survey found that women spend an average of $3,756 per year on beauty products and services, which is more than $10 a day.[34] Amongst younger generations, the figure can be even higher: women in their twenties report spending over $9,000 annually on beauty.[35] And it's not just about money – surveys suggest American women devote nearly an hour (55–60 minutes) per day to appearance-related activities, much of that dedicated to make-up application.[36]

These statistics represent millions of daily rituals and billions of individual decisions, all taking place within an industry built on the underlying belief that our natural faces require improvement.

The History of Make-Up

To understand make-up's grip on our modern psyche, we need to dig deeper than current TikTok and YouTube tutorials and explore its origin. Because make-up is far from a new phenomenon: it's one of humanity's oldest aesthetic rituals. Across continents and centuries, people have used different kinds of pigments, powders and pastes to alter how the face appears, and what's evolved over time is not the underlying desire to alter appearance, but the tools, the scales, the motivation and the stakes.

From ancient Egyptian times (as early as 4,000 BCE) men and women alike lined their eyes with kohl made from ground galena (lead sulfide) or malachite – they not only believed that it enhanced their beauty but also that it warded off evil spirits and protected their eyes from the harsh desert glare. They used red ochre to tint lips and cheeks, while scented oils were used as both skincare and a sign of status. Make-up was more than a means of looking good; it was tied to health, religion and power.

In Mesopotamia, a region in Iraq, women crushed semi-precious stones to decorate their lips and eyes, while in ancient Greece, white lead was used to achieve a pale, smooth complexion associated with wealth and leisure. Greek women also applied ground cinnabar to their cheeks and lips, despite its toxic mercury content. Rome embraced similar ideals, with women lightening their skin using chalk or lead carbonate and tinting their cheeks with red iron oxide. A pale complexion signalled class privilege: it implied you were wealthy enough to avoid outdoor labour. Already, at this early point in history, a pattern was beginning to emerge, with cosmetics acting as class markers, and a specific type of beauty (namely, whiteness) being perceived as the ultimate sign of attractiveness.

During the Tang dynasty in China (618–907 CE), make-up reached new heights: women powdered their faces with rice flour, painted delicate flower patterns on their cheeks and blackened their eyebrows into carefully shaped arches. Meanwhile, in Japan's Heian period (794–1185 CE), women in the royal court made white rice-powder faces fashionable, along with ohaguro, the practice of blackening their teeth.

By the Elizabethan era in England, the beauty ideal for pale skin remained – this time, achieved from ceruse, a deadly mix of white lead and vinegar. Rouge for cheeks and lips came from plant dyes or cochineal insects and women sometimes painted on blue veins to enhance the impression of translucent, 'aristocratic' skin. Hairlines were plucked back to elongate the forehead, demonstrating the way in which beauty practices have long involved embellishing *and* reshaping the body.

The eighteenth century saw both men and women in European aristocracy embracing highly stylised make-up: thick white powder and bright rouge, with many even donning stickers cut into heart or star shapes – not unlike the Star Face patches we see today. The looks were theatrical and deliberately conspicuous, reinforcing class divides. Cosmetics were expensive, messy and often toxic and their wearers were signalling status by using them.

A backlash against make-up emerged in the Victorian era, with heavy cosmetics becoming associated with sex work and moral corruption, prompting 'respectable' women to adopt subtle methods of beautification like homemade skin creams, discreet lip tints and natural-looking powders. The emphasis shifted to looking naturally beautiful while still investing time and effort into maintaining that appearance – a dynamic that still exists today.

It was in the twentieth century that make-up transformed into mass consumer culture. The rise of photography, cinema and, later, television created new pressures to appear 'camera-ready'. Max Factor Sr., a Polish-born American make-up artist and businessman, is credited with coining the noun 'make-up' when he launched a consumer cosmetics line in the 1920s and 1930s. He revolutionized the industry by producing formulas like Pan-Cake foundation, a lightweight, all-in-one product still widely used today, and helped transform make-up from theatrical craft into everyday beauty tool. Post-war brands like Revlon and Maybelline, meanwhile, tapped into emerging mass media and advertising to sell products and ideas like glamour, modernity and self-expression. Make-up became synonymous with aspiration and identity.

By the 1960s, celebrity icons like Twiggy and Brigitte Bardot helped amplify this cultural shift. Twiggy, dubbed 'The Face of 1966', established an iconic 'mod' look defined by oversized eyes accentuated with heavy liner, dramatic lower lashes (often drawn on with liner) and white liner to enlarge and brighten the eye area. Brigitte Bardot, the French film star, popularised bold winged liner.

The decades that followed saw make-up styles evolve alongside social change, music and media. In the 1970s, the influence of disco and glam rock brought glittery eyeshadows, frosted lipsticks and a more playful, experimental approach to colour. At the same time, the growing feminist movement sparked debate about make-up's role – whether it was an oppressive tool of the patriarchy or a form of self-expression that women could reclaim on their own terms (a conversation we are, clearly, *still* having today!). The 1980s dialled everything up: bold blush, vivid eyeshadow and power lipstick reflected an era preoccupied with excess and confidence.

Minimalism took centre-stage in the 1990s: nude lips, matte skin and neutral eyeshadows dominated runways, influenced by the rise of supermodels like Kate Moss and the 'heroin chic' aesthetic, much as it pains me to even type the phrase. The 2000s flipped things again, embracing shimmer, gloss, bronzer and highly stylised brows, driven by celebrity culture, reality TV and red-carpet beauty.

By the 2010s, social media and YouTube 'beauty gurus' had transformed make-up into both a global industry machine, complete with contouring tutorials, make-up haul videos and influencer collaborations. At the heart of this shift was the enormous influence of Kim Kardashian, whose highly stylised, full-glam looks – flawless base, heavy concealer, heavy contour, sharp brows, false lashes, bold shiny highlighter and overlined lips – set the beauty template for an entire decade. She helped make contouring a household term and turned beauty routines into hour-long, multi-step processes.

Kim's sister, Kylie Jenner, began selling lip kits in 2015 – they frequently sold out within minutes and grew into a billion-dollar beauty brand, proving that influencer-led make-up lines could rival long-established cosmetic houses. This direct-to-consumer model, driven by social media hype, changed the way beauty was sold forever. Make-up trends could now be created, copied and discarded in a matter of weeks, and the pressure to be and stay 'on trend' intensified.

By the early 2020s, the pendulum began to swing away from heavy contour and full glam towards a much softer, more minimalist ideal – the 'clean girl' aesthetic. Popularised on TikTok and Instagram by influencers like Hailey Bieber and Matilda Djerf, this look emphasised dewy skin, brushed-up blows, glossy lips and barely-there make-up that appeared effortless, yet still required a curated selection of products: skin tints, cream blushes, cream bronzers, highlighter drops, brow gels, lip oils. It was marketed as low-maintenance, but in practice it relied on the same underlying perfectionism as the full-glam era, just presented in subtler packaging.

Make-Up Today

I'm writing this towards the end of 2025, and it looks like bold beauty is making its return: rich berry tones, neon lashes, eye-catching eyeliner and unapologetically colourful looks. The make-up industry is now worth over $76 billion a year.[37]

Make-up trends, just like fashion, have always moved in cycles. What changes isn't the impulse to enhance, but the speed at which the industry can package, sell and discard each look – especially in today's world of social media. In the past, it might have taken years for a style to trickle down from catwalk to the make-up counter, but now TikTok can take a product from obscurity to sold out worldwide in less than 48 hours.

It's also important to acknowledge that these trends are more than purely aesthetic shifts; they're also economic strategies. Every swing of the trend pendulum creates a new set of 'must have' products. The global make-up market thrives on constant reinvention, conditioning us to see last year's look as outdated and this season's as essential. It's a template that can be copied and pasted directly from the fashion industry.

The through-line throughout history is clear: make-up has always been about more than 'looking pretty'. It reflects beliefs about class, gender, wealth and power. Its materials may have shifted from ground minerals and poisonous lead (thank goodness!) to high-tech, long-wear formulas, but its role as both a tool of self-expression and a means of conformity remains remarkably constant.

There's a reason why so many of us laugh in recognition when *The Guilty Feminist* host Deborah Frances-White quips: 'I'm a feminist – but I would rather cancel a date than show up without eyeliner.' Because going without make-up still feels transgressive, even risky. The joke lands because it captures a very real tension: we can know the politics, we can believe in equality and yet we can still feel tethered to make-up in ways that don't always sit comfortably with our values.

So, maybe the question isn't, 'Is make-up feminist?', it's: 'How do we navigate our relationship with it honestly?'

Truly, I'm not sure I really have the answer myself, and that uncertainty makes me, by some definitions, a hypocrite. I call myself a feminist, I know the mechanics of how beauty culture works, I can spot the marketing manipulations a mile away – and yet, most days, I still won't leave the house without mascara and concealer.

But I think that's where I have to sit right now. Hypocrisy is, in some ways, inevitable when you're trying to live authentically inside a system you can't fully opt out of. We're all negotiating compromises between our politics, our pleasures and our survival. Pretending otherwise – pretending that there's a perfect, ideologically pure way to move through the world – feels dishonest and somewhat unrealistic (at least for me).

Maybe the point isn't to be untouched by the system, but to stay conscious inside it. To notice when our choices are driven by joy and when they're driven by fear. To interrogate those moments without shaming ourselves for them. And to remember that resisting beauty norms doesn't always have to mean abandoning beauty altogether – sometimes it's about reshaping the meaning of it, on our own terms.

The Headlines
- Make-up has long existed in the tension between self-expression and self-surveillance
- The beauty industry relies on a cycle of insecurity and reinvention, turning trends into profit and conditioning us to view our natural features as 'before' states in need of fixing
- Make-up functions differently for different people: for some it's art, for some it's armour and for some it's a multitude of things – and all of those are OK
- Gender, class and race all inform how and why people wear make-up
- The pressure to appear 'polished' or 'professional' through wearing make-up is very real: research shows that make-up materially affects how women are perceived, hired and valued
- Ultimately, our relationship with make-up is shaped by both personal desire and cultural conditioning, and it is arguably almost impossible to untangle these two forces completely.

A Moment of Reflection
- *When did I first learn that a bare face was something to apologize for – and who taught me that?*
- *What emotions come up for me when I imagine going out without make-up: freedom, fear, indifference, vulnerability?*
- *How often do I wear make-up because I want to – and how often because I worry about how I'll be perceived without it?*
- *Which beauty choices feel aligned with my identity, and which feel like a performance for others?*
- *Who benefits when I doubt my natural appearance? And who benefits when I feel connected to joy, play and self-expression instead?*

Where Do We Go From Here?

I don't think we need to decide whether make-up is good or bad, feminist or anti-feminist. I think we can acknowledge that it can be both, and that our relationship with it deserves respect, not judgement.

It's almost impossible to fully step outside a culture that treats beauty as currency, but we *can* become more conscious. We can notice the moments when we're acting from pressure rather than pleasure or choice and we can question the messages around our natural appearance that we inherited.

Make-up is complicated, and so are we. And I think there's real liberation in letting that complexity exist without shame.

Chapter 7

The Tweakment Trap

When I was in my late teens and early twenties, beauty maintenance looked very different. Apart from regularly attacking my eyebrows with tweezers (a rite of passage for any self-respecting millennial, and one that we're still paying for with sparse patches), I might get my nails done as a treat every now and again, or maybe I'd fake tan before a night out (Sally Hansen Airbrush Legs, anyone?!), but regular eyebrow appointments, lash extensions, spray tans, facials or tweakments weren't part of my routine. Going to a professional for a treatment felt like a luxury – indulgences reserved for special occasions, rather than an expectation. In the early 2000s, Botox and filler were only whispered about. They were the preserve of the rich and famous, framed as drastic interventions, and they certainly weren't part of the everyday language of beauty.

Fast forward to today and the landscape has shifted dramatically. Invasive beauty treatments have moved into the mainstream, so much so that many perceive them as standard upkeep, integral to self-care. They are widely available – you can now find aesthetic clinics on almost every high street and even in mainstream stores like Superdrug – and marketed as sitting alongside haircuts, manicures and gym memberships as part of routine self-care and 'maintenance', or even 'preventative' treatments. The question is less 'Do you get anything done?' and more '*What* do you get done?'

The Rise of Tweakments

Today, the menu of options for 'self-improvement' is dizzying: Botox; filler; skin boosters; lip flips; under-eye brightening; chin sculpting; tear trough filler; baby Botox; Barbie Botox; masseter Botox; salmon sperm injections; thread lifts; brow lifts; fox eye lifts; buccal fat removal; lip blushing; microblading; 'vampire' facials; microneedling; chemical peels; dermaplaning; mesotherapy; cryotherapy facials; LED light therapy; IV drips; collagen stimulators; exosome therapy; fat-dissolving injections . . . you get the point. The baseline of 'normal' beauty upkeep has shifted drastically and the rise of tweakments is one of the clearest indicators of its speed and progression.

The data backs up this sentiment. Back in the early 2000s, Botox had only just been approved for cosmetic use and was marketed almost exclusively to older women with disposable income. Cosmetic procedures were a niche industry, worth around $24 billion globally in 2005.[38] Today, the market is measured in tens of billions worldwide, with non-surgical procedures driving much of the growth forecasts towards well over $60-70 billion by the early 2030s.[39] In the UK, non-invasive treatments such as Botox and filler grew by 15 per cent in a single year – 2024 – contributing more to the economy than sport and live entertainment combined.[40]

The cultural shift is just as striking. In 2022, more than half of women surveyed said they had tried a non-surgical procedure for the first time within the past year, and 81 per cent said these treatments are now far more acceptable than five years ago.[41] These procedures are now seen less as drastic changes than as subtle interventions – just enough to look refreshed, polished and 'naturally' beautiful.

The goal, now, is not to look radically different. Rather, it's to look like yourself – but *better*. It's an aesthetic that mirrors current cultural preferences: natural but curated; undone, but perfected; effortless, but expensive. You should look like you've had a full eight hours of sleep, been passed down impeccable genes, have a green juice habit and the blurring Instagram 'Paris' filter built into your face.

What's striking is the unsettling uniformity that's emerging from this: the 'natural' look has its own kind of template, with subtly plump lips, slightly lifted brows, poreless skin and softly contoured cheeks. It feels like the homogenisation of 'authenticity'. There's also something deeply gendered in the expectation that women should appear 'perfect' without appearing to have tried. Visible effort carries stigma and it's a deeply unfair expectation. We're told to 'age gracefully' but also to 'maintain ourselves' and it's a contradiction that keeps women treading a fine line. It's an exhausting but crystal-clear message – be beautiful, but don't let anyone see that you've worked for it.

This is a pivot from the more maximalist 2010s, when the

prevailing beauty template was the so-called 'Instagram Face': pillowy lips, sharp jawline, lifted brows, poreless matte skin. The mid-2010s were a perfect storm for cosmetic procedures: celebrity confessionals drove demand – Kylie's 2015 lip-filler reveal was followed by a reported 70 per cent surge in enquiries – and hyaluronic acid fillers were suddenly ubiquitous. By 2015, fillers were already being used by nearly two million people annually in the US, making them the second most popular non-surgical procedure after Botox; by 2019, soft-tissue fillers topped 2.5 million, up a staggering 300 per cent since 2000.[42]

Three things accelerated the growth of tweakments. First, the speed with which they can be acquired: 'lunchtime' procedures with minimal downtime slotted easily into people's lives. Secondly, the promise of reversibility: because most popular fillers are hyaluronic acid-based, clinics could sell a safety net – *if you hate it, we can dissolve it*. The most powerful accelerant was, of course, social media. Celebrities may have introduced tweakments to the mainstream, but platforms like Instagram and TikTok helped them explode in popularity.

The line between skincare and injectables began to blur, and TikTok, in particular, was instrumental in normalizing them. 'Get ready with me' videos and 'glow-up' transformations regularly detailed tweakments, positioning them as vital self-care. Influencers and reality stars slipped procedures into sponsored content, suggesting that tweakments were aspirational but attainable, and my own feed, like so many others, became crowded with split-screen videos advertising clinics: one side showing a celebrity who has 'taken care of herself' (read: had tweakments or plastic surgery) paired with one who 'hasn't'. These posts would often be accompanied by a smug caption suggesting it's our choice to decide which version we'd prefer to look like.

All this, combined with loose UK regulations that allow non-medical practitioners to deliver injectables, meant that as well as the glossy transformations, there were also horror stories. There were many who were unhappy with the results and, subsequently, there was a surge in 'fix' visits to correct botched procedures. In 2018 alone, Save Face, a Professional Standards Authority-accredited register that inspects clinics and practitioners, and publishes complaint data, logged 934 adverse reports, around two-thirds of which were tied to fillers.[43] These numbers prompted years of clamouring for tighter rules and regulations around the procedures.

By the late-2010s, tweakments were booming. Then came the pandemic. Lockdowns might have temporarily caused clinics to close, but the endless video calls created new neuroses born out of staring at our own faces, day after day, under 'unflattering' lighting and odd camera angles. Unlike looking in a mirror, which is fleeting and intentional, online meetings forced us into a constant state of self-surveillance. Every wrinkle, every fine line, uneven skin tone and even the tiniest bit of asymmetry was magnified.

Dermatologists and psychologists called it 'Zoom dysmorphia', and when clinics reopened, pent-up demand collided with these amplified insecurities. Enquiries skyrocketed, with the British Association of Aesthetic Plastic Surgeons reporting a 70 per cent increase in requests for cosmetic procedures after the first lockdown. US dermatologists saw similar spikes, with some practices reporting 50 per cent more demand than before the pandemic.[44]

Yet, as demand soared, a new unease began to creep in and by the early 2020s the overfilled look was losing its sheen and fast heading towards a PR problem. 'Pillow face' – a look associated with excess filler in the face – became a meme, and on TikTok 'filler migration' videos, showing how product can drift beyond its intended area, racked up millions of views. More unnerving still, new imaging studies started showing that so-called 'temporary' hyaluronic acid in fillers can remain in the body for years – often far beyond the marketed 6–12 months. Our collective desire for filler injections had finally started to wane.

Celebrities and influencers began publicly backtracking, too: Courteney Cox spoke about dissolving her filler; *Love Island*'s Molly-Mae Hague documented having hers dissolved; and even Kylie Jenner experimented with more natural proportions. The tide was turning: the 'Instagram Face' era was out; the 'natural but better' aesthetic was in.

Eventually, regulators started to catch up, and finally stepped in. In 2020, the UK's ad watchdog reminded clinics and influencers that you can't market prescription-only toxins like Botox to the public on social media. Thousands of posts were flagged and removed, but despite the crackdown, a 2023 *Guardian* article noted that nine out of ten beauty clinics were still breaking the law by advertising Botox and other forms of botulinum toxin. The Health and Care Act of 2022 paved the way for new licensing schemes for non-surgical cosmetic procedures and, in August 2025, the government published new, tighter standards for who can inject, where, and under what safeguards. Under-eighteens were also excluded from treatments.

With the culture vigilant to obvious 'work', aesthetics pivoted to the new, more 'natural' era that is in play today. Smaller doses, skin 'boosters', collagen 'stimulators' and polynucleotides all began to be sold in the soothing language of 'skin health', with the new aim being to look permanently well-rested. The results are, of course, far less visible than the previous iteration, so you'd be forgiven for assuming that it might translate to less time, less money and less effort, but the truth is that the 'natural' look still demands a significant amount of all those things. The labour of beauty didn't vanish, unfortunately. Women are still expected to visit salons, spend precious time and money on multiple treatments and tweakments, just under the guise of 'maintenance' rather than 'transformation'.

Celebrities and Tweakments

Celebrity culture perfectly illustrates this shift. Take Lindsay Lohan, whose 2025 appearances sparked a frenzy of speculation about her 'new face'. For years, Lindsay had been relatively quiet on the Hollywood front, living in Dubai, raising her child and staying out of the relentless paparazzi spotlight. Then, almost overnight, at the age of 38, she stepped back onto the red carpet and into interviews looking noticeably different. I don't want to add to the speculation by, well, speculating myself, but let's just say she looked fresher, smoother and more polished than the version many remembered from her twenties and early thirties.

The reaction was instant. 'She's ageing in reverse,' one TikTok user commented. 'I will pay any amount of money to have this done to my face, she looks STUNNING,' said another. Social media lit up with split-screen comparisons of her past and present looks. TikTok doctors, dermatologists and plastic surgeons posted forensic-like breakdowns of her face, zooming in on her jawline, cheeks and under-eyes, offering theories about what procedures she had done: mini facelift? Morpheus8? Threads? Laser resurfacing? Botox and filler in carefully measured doses? Some praised her for 'ageing backwards', while others insisted it was 'too much work too young' or accused her of being 'vain'.

Why the frenzy? It's common knowledge by now that many celebrities utilise plastic surgery and tweakments, but the excitement was perhaps in part due to Lindsay having been out of the spotlight: there was no gradual drip-feed of change through constant paparazzi images, making the contrast stark. The timing also played a role: by 2025, we were deep in the era of the 'natural-but-expensive' look. Lindsay perfectly embodied this new aesthetic, so naturally, everyone wanted to know her secret recipe. In an interview with *Elle*, she pushed back against the facelift rumours with a joke – 'When? With what time? Where?' – but admitted openly to Botox, 'Everyone does Botox', and treatments like lasers and Morpheus8, a cosmetic treatment that combines microneedling with radiofrequency energy to tighten skin, stimulate collagen and 'contour' the face or body.

I must be honest here: Lindsay Lohan's 'glow-up' got under my skin (pun intended). Lindsay and I are roughly the same age (she was born in 1986, while I was born in 1988) and as the internet pored over her face, I couldn't help but compare myself. For a few fleeting moments, I found myself wondering whether I should be doing something too: *Should I be preserving, preventing, correcting? Would I benefit from lifting my brows? Do my eyes droop?*

I suddenly felt a crushing pressure in a way I never had before. I was overwhelmed by the sense that even at my age of 36, my face had already become a project that required intervention. It was a quick spiral: a split-screen video of Lindsay on my feed, a stray glance in the mirror, and suddenly I was running a comprehensive audit of my own features and my perceived flaws. That moment passed, but it left its mark. It showed me how easy it is to be pulled into the undercurrent of comparison, even as someone who spends her life questioning beauty standards. It also demonstrated how powerful the cultural expectation has become: that to be seen, and to be admired, is to appear untouched by time. I can't even begin to imagine how it feels for women older than me.

Lindsay isn't an outlier; she's part of a much bigger pattern – the cycle of obsession and speculation that emerges when women reach midlife. Demi Moore is another case in point: in 2025, the actress found herself in the centre of an appearance-based frenzy after a string of public appearances where she was looking, perhaps, younger than she had previously. TikTok and YouTube were inundated with side-by-side breakdowns of her looks throughout the 1990s, 2010s and 2025, each frame dissected with precision. Some praised her for looking 'amazing for her age', while others accused her of looking 'unnatural' and criticized her for 'not ageing gracefully' – a euphemism for having work done.

The 'Battle' Against Ageing

The phrase 'ageing gracefully' sounds flattering, but really, it's just another form of control for women. It implies that there's a correct way to age: visibly, but attractively; natural, but not *too* natural; older, but never *old*. It's a demand to maintain beauty while pretending not to care about it and it is a double standard that men are simply not subjected to.

But back to Lindsay: plastic surgeons and aesthetic influencers churned out endless 'what has she had done?' videos, often with millions of views, and the fixation was so intense that the speculation about her appearance often drowned out coverage of her actual projects. Demi herself has never confirmed or denied specific procedures, but her silence hasn't shielded her. If anything, it has made her more of a blank canvas onto which everyone can project their assumptions. Clinics even used her images in Instagram posts as a kind of free marketing to demonstrate how effective tweakments can be.

This cycle isn't one that Demi Moore, Lindsay Lohan, or any other woman in the public eye can opt out of. Whether she denies it, admits it or says nothing at all, her face will, nevertheless, be treated as public property. The reason for this is our unrelenting desire for answers. We are desperate to know how it's possible for anyone to stay youthful, natural and flawless when the standard itself is designed to be impossible. The endless speculation doesn't just land on the celebrity at the heart of it, either; it lands on us mere mortals, too, leaving us feeling that we are constantly chasing a standard we never agreed to, let alone one that we stand a chance of reaching.

If Lindsay Lohan and Demi Moore show us what happens when women do opt to undergo some form of intervention, Sarah Jessica Parker shows us what happens when they don't. The *Sex and the City* actress's decision to age 'naturally' has been met with relentless and often cruel backlash, with a wealth of scathing, ageist commentary both online and in the press. It's the perfect illustration of the bind women constantly find themselves in – damned if we do, damned if we don't. Intervene, and you're mocked for vanity; resist, and you've 'let yourself go'.

The idea of ageing naturally here doesn't necessarily mean that Sarah Jessica Parker does nothing at all – she's spoken about going to dermatologists, having facials and using treatments like peels and lasers, but she's also talked about resisting the more heavy-handed interventions like Botox and filler that many of her peers adopt. She's also allowed her hair to turn grey, and this light-touch approach to beauty makes her stand out in an industry where 'maintenance' is increasingly a code word for injectables, surgery and endless hours of hidden labour.

It's so telling that this choice not to partake in the machine of anti-ageing sparks such fury. Sarah Jessica Parker's refusal to erase the visible signs of the passing of time is treated less as an individual choice and more as a provocation. When paparazzi shots of her grey hair circulated in 2021, the internet erupted with derision, prompting her to call out the 'misogynist chatter' that would never be directed at a man. 'Grey hair, grey hair, grey hair. Does she have grey hair?' she said to *Vogue*. 'I'm sitting with Andy Cohen, and he has a full head of grey hair, and he's exquisite. Why is it OK for him?'

This is an excellent point – and one we'll get onto shortly – but SJP had more to say about the impossible bind that women face: 'She has too many wrinkles. She doesn't have enough wrinkles. It almost feels as if people don't want us to be perfectly OK with where we are, as if they enjoy us being pained by who we are today ... I know what I look like. I have no choice. What am I going to do about it? Stop ageing? Disappear?'

These words feel spot on. We live in a culture that derives satisfaction from policing women's bodies at every turn, and Sarah Jessica's refusal to morph into a cosmetic ideal, and the subsequent discourse around that decision, shows how little room there is for women to simply exist without being turned into a moral lesson about ageing.

Taken together, these three examples reveal the trap at the heart of beauty culture: there is no way to 'win'. Compliance doesn't grant women freedom; it only reshapes the scrutiny. Women who pursue tweakments are labelled vain, frivolous or self-obsessed, while women who resist are branded as 'careless' or accused of 'letting themselves go'. Either way, the judgement sticks.

The trickle-down effect is that celebrity faces become templates for how the rest of us measure our own, magnifying insecurities and fuelling the sense that we, too, are being perceived and judged at every turn. Lindsay and Demi's 'new faces'; Sarah Jessica's grey hair – each becomes a cultural flashpoint, but the impact isn't confined to them. Instead, it seeps outwards, setting the terms by which every woman is judged and, more insidiously, by which we judge ourselves.

This is how celebrity culture functions – as a system of standards. When a red-carpet photo of Lindsay Lohan goes viral, the subtext isn't just, 'look at her', it's 'look at yourself'. Each of these women, along with the thousands who have come before, and those who will inevitably come after, are held up as evidence of what is possible and what is acceptable. All this results in a referendum on what the rest of us should be doing with our own faces.

The Mental Toll

Of course, in an ideal world, this wouldn't be the case. We wouldn't measure ourselves against celebrities whose lives, resources and access to treatments look nothing like our own. It's also worth considering that, for many of these women in the public eye, their appearance is not just about vanity but about currency: looking a certain way can determine whether they get cast, hired, endorsed or erased. In an ideal world, we wouldn't internalize their choices as verdicts on our own worth – instead, we would be free to live according to our own standards, deciding how we want to show up in the world without the constant hum of comparison.

The sad truth is that humans don't work that way; we're wired for comparison. Evolution taught us to scan others as a way of locating ourselves in the group: it was once a matter of survival. Today, that instinct plays out in subtler ways: we compare careers, relationships, bodies, homes, even happiness, and all of this is supercharged by social media, which essentially puts a global pageant in the palm of our hands, 24/7. Instead of existing outside of beauty standards, we find ourselves pulled into them, whether we agree with them or not. Whilst we may rationally know that the reaction to Lindsay Lohan's 'new face' or Sarah Jessica Parker's grey hair has nothing to do with our own value, the cultural script is powerful enough that it still seeps into how we feel about our own reflection.

'Appearance anxiety' is a term coined by psychologists to describe the persistent worry or distress someone feels about how they look, whether it's their weight, skin, hair, ageing or any other aspect of their appearance. It's not the same as wanting to look nice for a night out, for example – this goes far deeper and is representative of something more chronic. It could involve mentally replaying which aspects of your appearance others might have noticed, avoiding certain social settings because of how you think you'll be perceived, or constantly comparing yourself to others. Appearance anxiety creates a sense that your face and body are an ongoing project with no clear finish line, and it takes a huge toll.

That's where the promise of tweakments slips in so seductively. They're marketed as the solution to the constant burden of self-consciousness; a way to silence the noise by 'fixing' whatever flaw keeps you up at night. These procedures may appear to be empowering you to take charge of how you look on your own terms, and to stay one step ahead of time itself. The reality is that they end up controlling us: our money, our calendars, our headspace. They leave women feeling permanently unfinished, always searching for the next tweak or the next procedure that might finally make us feel 'enough'.

Still worse, these treatments are packaged as 'leisure'; something that shouldn't take much of a toll. Just a top-up appointment here, and a ten-step skincare routine there – it's all framed as self-care; small acts of empowerment that are our choice. In reality, though, it's relentless work. The researching, the booking, the mental toll, the paying, the justifying. And even when we do comply, the goalposts for how we should look move yet again.

The Freedom to Choose

I want to be clear that none of this is about shaming women for choosing tweakments. I'm also not declaring them to be inherently bad. Women should be free to do whatever they want with their faces and bodies. If Botox, filler, lasers or any other kind of tweakment makes someone feel more comfortable in their own skin, that's their prerogative – and in many ways, it is a completely understandable response to a culture that frames ageing as a failure.

I certainly feel the pressure, and I've dabbled with Botox myself. I hated the way that it made me feel 'better'. That single word carried so much judgement about my unaltered face, as if my natural state had been lacking all along; the 'before' to fix. I was also concerned that it would quickly become a slippery slope – if smoothing my forehead wrinkles made me feel better, what else would I start wanting to correct? Where would that logic end?

We are not the villains here, for having tweakments. The blame lies solely with the rigged system we're all forced to live inside; a culture that tells women our worth is conditional and that we can never quite be enough as we are.

This is why solidarity and compassion matter. Too often, women's choices about beauty get turned into battlegrounds: Botox vs 'ageing gracefully'. We end up judging each other for how we navigate the pressure, as if there is a right or wrong way to survive and thrive in a world where we're damned if we do and damned if we don't (spoiler alert: there isn't).

Instead of turning that scrutiny on one another, what if we redirected it to the system itself? What if the energy we spend debating who's done what went into asking why women are forced to justify their faces at all? Solidarity doesn't mean we all have to make the same choices; it means recognizing that every choice is made in an environment designed to make us feel insufficient. The real liberation isn't in picking a side, but in questioning why sides even exist in the first place.

The Economics of Tweakments

This is where economics come in, because the beauty industry isn't just a backdrop to these pressures; it's the engine driving it forward. It's no coincidence that the shame around ageing has been so effectively weaponised when the potential for profits is so huge. Our fear doesn't exist in a vacuum; it's been nurtured, marketed and sold back to us in pretty packaging, because the beauty industry is acutely aware of what ageing represents to women: an almost inevitable loss of visibility, value and power. And it knows exactly how to monetise that fear.

The global anti-ageing market is now worth an estimated $63 billion[45] – and it's growing. It spans creams, serums, lasers, facials, supplements, tweakments, surgeries, 'miracle' ingredients and double-digit-step skincare routines, all sold to us with the promise of making us look younger. Instead of getting older being presented as a life stage, it has become a condition; a visible threat that needs to be blurred, plumped, tightened, corrected – reversed, essentially – at any cost. We're taught to fight ageing, as if it's a battle we can win *if we just buy the right products*. Even the term 'anti-ageing' reveals a deeper truth: the industry is selling the idea that ageing is a failure, and that, to succeed, we must delay and disguise it for as long as possible.

Billions are made each year from women's insecurities – the business model quite literally depends on it. Tweakments are especially profitable because they create repeat customers. Botox wears off, filler dissolves, skin boosters need topping up. Each treatment is sold as progress, but it is progress that requires constant maintenance. When tweakments are framed less as luxury add-ons and more as routine necessities, opting out doesn't feel neutral anymore – it feels like neglect.

This economic engine doesn't operate in isolation – it's supported by a cultural ecosystem that makes resistance nearly impossible. Even if we consciously reject the pressure to look 25 forever, it doesn't mean we're immune to it. The images we're surrounded by still idealize youth; the beauty campaigns still quietly exclude older faces, and the compliments still hinge on looking younger than you are. Even our most progressive spaces – feminist, creative, inclusive – often still fail to centre or even *include* older women. As a result, women are left to navigate ageing alone, in a world that tells us that our worth declines with each birthday.

The Gender Gap

Here's the part that really stings (although I know this is all quite sting-y so far): the industry is designed to keep women locked into this cycle, while men are, largely, allowed the grace to simply age.

Now look, I don't want to be dismissive of men's experiences with beauty standards because I know that they, too, are subject to societal pressures. Nevertheless, these standards disproportionately impact women – and nowhere is this clearer than in the arena of ageing. Men age, and they gain charisma, along with adjectives like 'distinguished', 'seasoned', or 'silver fox'. Fine lines are read as experience. Men aren't sold 'maintenance' as a moral duty, and they're not told that grey hair or wrinkles are signs of neglect.

By contrast, women age and they gain assignments: fix it, hide it, apologize for it, erase it at all costs. Workplaces reinforce this double standard – ageing men become mentors and figures of authority, while ageing women become cautionary tales. He has 'gravitas', while she's 'brave for her age'. And dating follows the same script: a 55-year-old man with crow's feet is 'rugged', while a 55-year-old woman with identical lines 'looks good for her age' – a backhanded compliment at best.

Navigating Midlife

As we've already established, women are punished for compliance and punished for refusal. There is no winning position, only a permanent state of defence. And this is where the pressure feels sharpest. Because while ageing for women is a physical process, it's also a social shift – a moment when visibility starts to dim and expectations tighten, right around the time when we are, arguably, finally beginning to know ourselves most.

For many women, this shift is accompanied by the menopause. Despite being a universal experience for half of the population, menopause remains strangely invisible. It shows up occasionally in medical pamphlets or in whispered conversations, but rarely is it seen in pop culture or in the media, let alone in beauty advertising. In recent years, though, advocates like Davina McCall have pushed menopause into the spotlight, using documentaries and campaigns to challenge the silence and demand better education, medical support and recognition. They have helped reframe menopause, not as an ending, but as a powerful new stage of life – yet despite this progress, the beauty industry has been slow to follow.

The symptoms of menopause can be disorientating and all-consuming: weight gain, hot flashes, brain fog, night sweats, mood swings, lowered libido, among a whole host of other symptoms. The emotional toll can also be crushing. For many women, menopause represents saying goodbye to a version of themselves they didn't know they were still holding onto – the fertile, youthful, 'desirable' self.

This stage of midlife is rarely acknowledged in empowering ways, and as a result it can feel like an erasure of identity. Women are told to expect it quietly, manage it discreetly and emerge on the other side without complaint. But menopause isn't the end of womanhood. It's another shift, and it deserves to be witnessed with the same reverence we give to puberty, pregnancy and every other hormonal shift in a woman's life. As author and menopause advocate Dr Jen Gunter writes: 'Menopause is not a disease . . . It's a life stage.' What if, instead of seeing it as a loss of womanhood, it was seen as just that: a life stage that represented the beginning of a different kind of power?

This kind of reframing requires a cultural shift that feels almost impossible when we're surrounded by messages that tell us the opposite. We're continuously taught to fear ageing: in teen magazines, in film scripts, in the compliments that taper off in our thirties. 'Anti-ageing' is more than a skincare label; it's a worldview, a warning that whispers to us that we were more valuable before.

The result is disorientating. One minute you're praised for 'looking so young' and the next you're scanning your face for evidence of time. There's also the creeping sense of erasure – not just to potential suitors, but in advertising, in job interviews, in the media, in beauty campaigns . . . your presence becomes less assumed and your value becomes less visible to society. The more that invisibility creeps in, the more desperate we may become to claw it back through products and procedures.

It feels brutal and wholly unjust that women's confidence and worth has a clock on it, and the fact that it does tells us something crucial. This isn't just about beauty standards, but about power and control. The world wants women kept busy: spending, apologizing, organizing, maintaining, worrying. It's a highly effective method; if women are consumed with self-surveillance, then the energy that could be directed outward is turned inward, and our lives become smaller.

If all of this feels deliberate, it's because it probably is. The patriarchy benefits enormously from keeping women locked in this cycle. A culture that teaches us to police our faces and bodies is one that keeps us busy, compliant and distracted. When we're caught up in calorie-counting, booking appointments, topping up injectables and second-guessing our own reflections, we have less bandwidth to question power structures, demand equity or claim space.

Beauty culture is a control mechanism that neatly supports the status quo, which is why moving toward something freer feels both urgent and complicated. What if we started with a different premise entirely? What if, instead of seeing ageing as something to fight, delay, or apologize for, we reframed it as what it actually is: a privilege? We've been taught to see ageing as a loss, a steady slide away from relevance and visibility and beauty; from being wanted, listened to, or even noticed. But what if that story isn't true? What if ageing is not a decline, but rather, a wonderful expansion?

We live in a culture that frames youth as the pinnacle, but youth is not a finish line – it's merely a starting point. It is beautiful, of course, but so is all that comes after – all the growth and depth and wisdom that comes from a life well-lived. What if we stop seeing age as the opposite of beauty, and start seeing it as just another form of it?

Yes, our bodies change, our skin softens, sags and creases. We may feel slower, our hormones fluctuate and our reflection evolves. But every one of those changes is proof that we are still here. Still living, still breathing, still becoming.

We carry our laughter and our millions of smiles in our crow's feet; we carry our worry in the lines between our brows; we carry our grief, our resilience, our joy and our rage on our skin. The beauty industry tells us that it's all something to hide and erase, as if the ultimate goal is to look like nothing has ever happened to look like we haven't lived. But the point is: so much has happened – and yet we're still here.

Reframing ageing as a privilege starts with acknowledging that not everyone gets to do it. Some people don't get the chance to grow older; some bodies don't make it to midlife; to menopause; to grey hair and forehead creases and decades of perspective.

Embracing ageing may be the most radical act of self-acceptance we'll ever be asked to perform, because in a culture that profits from our discomfort, choosing to embrace the very thing we've been taught to erase is not passive. It has to be intentional and active; powerful, political and rebellious.

For this to become more than a mantra, though, we need support. We need to see ageing women not just as side characters in sitcoms or cautionary tales in the media, but as leaders, lovers, protagonists – people with lives just as rich and complex and meaningful as those in younger bodies. We need to see older women in magazines; on screens; on billboards; in boardrooms; in beauty campaigns. We need the world to reflect what many of us already know deep down: that life doesn't stop being meaningful or beautiful once we pass a certain number.

Despite the narrow ideals still dominating the mainstream, there are women pushing back who refuse to become invisible. Andie MacDowell walked the Cannes red carpet with her grey curls worn proudly, challenging the idea that grey hair is something to cover or 'fix'. Viola Davis put it best when she said: 'The privilege of a lifetime is being who you are.' Tracee Ellis Ross calls ageing an honour, speaking of it not as a decline but as growth. Frances McDormand accepted her Oscar bare-faced and unapologetic, helping to rewrite Hollywood beauty rules, and Paulina Porizkova shares unfiltered selfies and writes with unflinching honesty about grief, invisibility, and the pride, and pain, of growing older in public.

These women aren't necessarily 'perfect' in their pursuit of rejecting 'anti-ageing' – whatever 'perfect' means. Some have had Botox, and some conform to beauty standards in other ways – but they don't have to be perfect. They're visible, and visibility matters.

The more we see older women at the centre of campaigns and stories and of their own lives, the more we start to undo the myth and the belief that our value fades with time.

Representation is only part of the solution, though. Language is one of the quietest ways that bias shows up – and when it comes to ageing, the language we use reveals a lot about how we truly feel.

We praise women for 'not looking their age', as though ageing is something to flee rather than embody; we call older women 'spritely' or 'youthful' as compliments, but rarely 'sexy', 'powerful' or 'beautiful'. Even well-meaning phrases carry bias. 'You look great for your age' or 'Wow, you don't look 50' still implies there's a standard you're expected to fall short of. 'She's still got it' suggests it was supposed to be gone. All of this language shapes our perception of what's acceptable and what's worth aspiring to. It quietly reinforces the idea that youth is the ultimate goal.

Maybe we need to look at the way we speak about ageing, instead complimenting energy, presence, charisma, expression. What if 'you look like you' could become the highest form of praise?

These shifts in language and representation matter, but they're still just pieces of a much larger puzzle.

So, what else can we do?

I don't have all the answers, but I do know that it's imperative that shame is eliminated. And that it is replaced with compassion: compassion for ourselves when we feel the pressure; compassion for other women when they make different choices from our own; and compassion when we stumble, because none of us is immune to the pull of comparison.

What we can do is start noticing, start naming the pressures for what they are, start asking who profits from our self-doubt, and choosing, where we can, to redirect our energy toward things that expand our lives rather than shrink them. Sometimes that means saying no to the cycle: choosing to let the grey grow in, skipping the appointment or deciding that the time and money could be better spent elsewhere. And other times it may mean saying yes: booking the facial, getting the Botox, buying the cream that makes you feel a little more confident when you look in the mirror. We need to let go of the binary that says you either embrace ageing and 'do nothing' or you fight it with every injectable and product you can get your hands on. There's room for both. You can have Botox and still love your ageing self; you can get regular facials and still celebrate the wisdom that comes with every passing year. But I believe we must, at all times, have our eyes open to the wider, harmful systems at play and recognize that these choices don't exist in a vacuum. We can want to feel good in our skin and still be furious at the system that made it so difficult.

When we say no, we push back against the system that profits from our insecurities, even if only in small ways. When we say yes, we can still do it consciously, without swallowing the lie that youth and flawlessness are prerequisites for worth. I don't believe that the danger lies necessarily within the individual choices, but in believing that these choices are the *only* route to value as a woman. Holding both truths at once – that it's OK to participate, and it's OK to resist – is how we loosen the grip of shame.

And importantly, going back to compassion because I think it's one of the most important aspects of this entire conversation, we can back each other. Instead of tearing down another woman for what she has or hasn't done, we can remind each other that there is no 'right' way to move through a rigged system. Solidarity is resistance.

It's not perfect, it's not complete and it's certainly not easy, but it's a start.

The Headlines
- Tweakments have shifted from niche, whispered-about procedures to mainstream maintenance now framed as routine self-care
- The rise of injectables, lasers and 'skin health' treatments is driven by a beauty economy built on insecurity, comparison and repeat consumption
- Social media has hugely accelerated demand, normalizing tweakments and blurring the line between 'aspiration' and expectation
- Women are punished whether they intervene or not: they're criticized for 'doing too much' or 'not doing enough', revealing the impossible double bind at the heart of beauty culture
- Ageing for women is both physical and social; visibility declines just as expectations intensify, reinforcing a gendered double standard that men simply do not face
- The problem is not the individual and a woman's individual choices; it is the system that makes those choices feel compulsory and frames natural ageing as a moral failure

A Moment of Reflection

- *When did I first start to believe that my face was something to manage, correct or preserve?*
- *Have I wanted tweakments because they felt empowering, or because not having them felt risky?*
- *What emotions come up when I see before-and-after photos, celebrity 'glow-ups' or split-screen online comparisons?*
- *Do I judge myself more harshly for ageing than I do the people I love?*
- *How much time, money and mental space do I spend monitoring or improving my appearance, and who benefits from that investment?*
- *When I think about ageing, what fear sits underneath it: invisibility, irrelevance, loss of desirability or something else entirely?*
- *What would compassion for myself (and for other women) look like in the face of all this pressure?*

Where Do We Go From Here?

As with most of the topics that we've discussed in this book, I don't believe the answer has to be to completely reject tweakments. I think we can start with removing the morality from tweakments and allow ourselves to participate, opt out, change our minds and hold nuance without turning any of it into a character indictment.

We can also shift our focus away from self-surveillance and towards self-connection. Instead of constantly monitoring our faces for lines or signs of 'decline', we can pay attention to how we actually *feel* in our bodies and our lives.

Really importantly, we can question who benefits from our insecurity – and who benefits when we reclaim our time, money and attention.

But most importantly, we need to realize with absolute certainty that ageing isn't a failure. Ageing is evidence that we're living, and the more we honour that, the less power the beauty industry has over us.

Chapter 8

Over To You . . .

This journey began with my story, but it was never only mine. From the very beginning, you have shared your experiences with me: stories of struggle, small moments of triumph and progress, and the often brutal, complicated realities of living in a world that judges a body before it sees the person within.

All the stories you've shared have shaped me – in the beginning, when I felt desperately alone, they were a huge source of comfort. They reminded me, again and again, that none of us is truly alone in this. Our relationship with body image often feels like a private battle fought in isolation, but the reality is that it is a shared experience, and a cultural inheritance that we all carry in different ways. We might all experience it differently, but the weight of it is something we can recognize in one another.

So, this final chapter doesn't just belong to me; it belongs to you, too. To the people who have written to me late at night feeling desperate; to those who have confided in me when it didn't feel safe yet to tell anyone else; to those who are still wrestling with the mirror or the scales or trying to fight back against the relentless beauty standards our culture projects onto us.

I asked you to submit your stories for this book, and I received hundreds of responses, each one a window into someone's private struggle and strength. While word-count limitations will only allow me to share a handful here, I need you to know that every single story that landed in my inbox is important to me. Each one reminded me that behind every statistic about body dissatisfaction is a real person trying to navigate this complicated world.

What you're about to read is a collection of voices that matter deeply. These are not all glossy stories with neat resolutions or perfect acceptance, but they *are* stories of doubt and courage and heartbreak and resilience, and they are all evidence of the fact that while none of us chose this inheritance, we do get to choose how we move forward with it – together.

My hope is that in reading these words, you will feel some of what I've been privileged to feel receiving these stories: connection, solidarity and the reminder that change is never an individual pursuit. We move the needle when we refuse to carry shame in silence; when we speak, when we listen and when we hold one another up.

So, without further ado, over to you . . .

Over To You . . .

Wendy, 42

I don't even know where to start. I have always been skinny to the point where my grandma would always say I looked like a lollipop stick – she always measured the thickness of my arms with her hand, saying, 'Oh my God, you need to eat more.' I had no fat, no boobs, no bum. I was bullied at school for being too skinny and boys laughed at me because I didn't wear a bra at thirteen. Bear in mind this is over twenty-five years ago. I never thought anything of it. Just normal banter. Well, was it?!

When I hit nineteen, I moved to England (I'm from Eastern Europe) and never really thought about my weight or looks. That wasn't a thing back then. I started to gain weight, you know, getting older, being on the pill, being in love, and I just noticed myself getting bigger. Around the same time, Facebook started, and obviously people began posting photos of themselves and you start to compare yourselves. That's where my first diet started. Dukan. I was even their 'Dukan Girl' for a while. I lost lots of weight, loved the comments on my Facebook posts and just enjoyed fitting in my clothes. Was I hungry and angry? Yes. Was I loving how I looked? Yes. This went on and off, because, as with any diet, once you stop, it just piled on. But I couldn't eat bloody ham and one gherkin for breakfast any longer. Yuck.

This went on for a while – I would be dieting in January, lose weight, feel happy, then gain it back, feel depressed, then diet. It was a vicious circle. I even went on two TV shows to lose weight, though watching them now, I see I wasn't even big! I did all the diets out there. Slimming World was bloody tough, especially the groups that made you feel guilty about gaining a pound.

Two years ago, I was about to hit forty, and that year, in January, I was thinking, *Crap, I need to go on a diet to look good for my fortieth*. But I didn't. I have no idea why, I just didn't. I went on holiday to Florida, where I took videos and photos and realized that I don't need to study how I look or check all my lumps, bumps, wrinkles. I was on holiday, with my husband, feeling great, and life is too short to care about such stupid things. I posted a video on my Instagram about hitting forty – and I loved it. I love how happy I look, even with chubby legs and stomach! I am sorry it took me so long to stop caring so much and say to myself: *take that photo, because you never know how long you have on this earth and what you see is different to what others see.*

Actually, while writing this I had a memory – in 2019, I did an advert for LinkedIn (I'm not a model, they needed real people) and I HATED the photos. I had no say in what would be used and my picture ended up on posters, buses, the Tube. But one of my friends sat me down and asked, 'What do you not like?' I said, *All of it: the double chin, the smile, the wrinkles around my eyes. All of it.* And she said, 'But that's you! You are gorgeous, and this is you. That picture is what everyone sees, but they don't see your double chin or wrinkles.' And at that moment I said to myself, *Yeah, that's how I look, this is me.* It was weird, but from then on, I looked at the photo as an outsider and not me judging it. That girl on that poster is gorgeous. And I share these photos because I *am* gorgeous.

OVER TO YOU . . .

Do I have bad days? Yes. Do I cry when I can't fit into my clothes? Yes. Do I sometimes get jealous of skinny people? Yes. But I don't hate me anymore. I am forty-two and recently started my TikTok – three years ago you would not get me in front of a camera! Now I'm constantly talking on camera and doing it for fun – not for views. I even wear leggings now! That is a BIG step up for me!

Amy, 32

Looking back, now that I have really come to love my body and all it can do, I truly cannot believe how much I hated my body, especially going through high school. I would be sick with anxiety about going to school because I truly couldn't understand why anyone would like me. Going to the beach, I would always be in long shorts and a T-shirt because I was embarrassed of my stomach and legs. It definitely got worse when Instagram became more popular, and I cared so much about how anything posted online would look. I wasn't bullied by anyone externally, but I felt a lot bigger than a lot of the girls I was friends with. I look back at photos, and I had nothing to worry about, but at the time it really felt like everything to me.

A few years ago, I really got bored of feeling like this and decided to spend less time online and really focused on finding a style that fit me. I was definitely hiding behind clothes, and since finding outfits that I really love (and not just focusing on clothes that make me smaller), I feel so much more confident. Objectively, I am now bigger than I was at school (obviously – I am an adult now), but I look forward to summer so I can wear my cute shorts and skirts and spend time at the beach in my bikini.

This has all been great for my self-esteem, the joy I feel in everyday life, but it really has made a huge positive improvement in my relationship. My husband always thought I looked amazing, but it's been wonderful for him to see me feeling that way too. We are going out more and laughing more, and I am so happy

Over To You . . .

with how far I have come from feeling like I was going to be ill every morning before school.

I really believe that cutting back on my social media use (and following positive accounts like yours) has helped along my body image journey.

Anonymous, 40

I am 40 years old, and my eating disorder started in my mid-late teens, with dieting and exercising to lose weight from a body that I felt conscious was 'not thin enough to be acceptable'. This was the 1990s, where there was basically zero representation of any body type other than 'very thin' – at least, none that were considered desirable, and I think that the combination of the media, fatphobia in my family and amongst my peers, alongside a vulnerability that already existed in me for various reasons, made me a prime candidate for developing an eating disorder. I battled with restriction, bingeing and purging until I went to have some in-patient treatment when I was 28. This was an extremely intense and surreal experience, none of it good by any means, but what I did learn in the three months I spent there was what it felt like to eat three meals and three snacks a day, and that it felt OK. I still struggled for a long time after treatment, but as I entered my thirties, a different kind of messaging was in the ether and creeping into my awareness. Body positivity, body neutrality, fat acceptance, intuitive eating . . . the algorithm was, for once, working in my favour, and I started to discover a world where people were not only letting go of trying to change their bodies but also to find some kind of peace with them, and with food and exercise.

I had retrained to become an integrative psychotherapist, having been a teacher all through my twenties, and I decided to do the Intuitive Eating Counsellor training course which was so helpful on both a personal and a professional level. It was the last piece of the puzzle for me. I had worked out that restricting my food caused me to binge, and making peace with food – i.e., that there are no good or bad ones – was a game-changer. I didn't feel guilt, shame and despair when I ate a carb; on the contrary, I knew I was doing something wonderfully healing and nourishing for my body. My weight settled somewhere in the middle of the extremes it had been at, which were not particularly extreme, by most people's standards, I realize now, and I have had a number of years of relatively peaceful eating and exercising.

There have been struggles – days, weeks or even months where things haven't felt OK – but I have managed to hold on and wait for them to pass without trying to do anything to 'fix' it, and have let my body move about in response when it has needed to, buying new clothes, dressing comfortably, practising self-compassion hard, and focusing on what I can do in my body, because it has survived such a horrendous illness.

Recent times things have felt more difficult. Although I have been working alongside registered dietitians for some years now to provide counselling for people on their own body image and disordered eating journey, the shift back to the 'thin ideal' has felt, quite frankly, depressing as shit. I have had to dig in a little harder with my own relationship with these things and, as a result, step back a little from the work and focus on other types of clients for the time being. I know, though, that it hasn't been for nothing. I would have had no defence against this current climate without the work that you do, and the work that I have done, and without the whole world that I discovered where people are given permission to eat, be in their bodies, rest and exist.

I know that fads pass; that Ozempic isn't a silver bullet; that it hasn't really 'changed' anything from my perspective, and that everyone needs to work out their own journey, in their own way and in their own time. What we have now, that can never be undone, is the knowledge that there *is* another way. As hard as it can be to do, and as hard as it can feel, we do not have to spend our lives trying to make ourselves smaller and sacrificing our happiness and health in the process. That's the choice I make today, and that I plan to make again tomorrow.

Over To You...

Steph, 32

I wanted to share my body image journey with you.

It started far too young. I was always heavier than my older sister, so my family took that and ran with it. When I was 6, I would eat an adult meal from Burger King and then finish my older sister's kid's meal. My uncle thought it was hilarious, so he took us out for it more often to get a quick laugh, I suppose. However, as I gained weight, his nickname for me turned into 'Chunks', which is something a child should never have to experience, and it's something I've carried with me for thirty-two years of life. I was never what doctors or society would even classify as overweight or obese, but in my mind, because of the environment I was living in, I was.

My mother, who was always a smaller woman, would constantly poke fun at my breast size because they were substantially larger than hers, which later caused me to be extremely self-conscious of them, something I never had any control of.

Fast forward to the age of twenty-four – I got Invisalign and that caused me to lose weight. Taking off those invisible braces to eat was so painful that I stopped snacking or drinking sugary drinks. I went from 160 lb to 115 lb in a few short months. And at that time, the compliments came in fast and furious. I almost felt like I was on a high because these comments and compliments had never come my way before. Even after my braces were done, I dove headfirst into restrictive eating. I said I hated French fries, even though I didn't. I'd drink my coffee black to avoid any calories. I'd count everything that went into my mouth.

Two years ago, my husband and I found out we were expecting.

It was a whirlwind. We wanted it so badly, but then the weight came on, and fast. I found myself eating everything, and there were points I wanted to throw it up because I felt so ashamed, before I realized I couldn't. I cried more about gaining weight than anything, and I hated being pregnant because of it. My body image issues ruined my pregnancy journey. I feel robbed of the experience.

Then, nine months later, my baby boy came into this world, and with thanks to you, Em Clarkson, Sarah Landry and all you incredible women, I was forced to realize bodies are *meant* to change. We did something absolutely incredible. I made, birthed and fed a human being. My body isn't something that's ruined now, it's something that's *made*. It's been made into a work of art because of the work of art I created, that little human that walks the earth because of what I did.

Thanks to you and your work, it's like a switch got flipped inside me, and I've never been more grateful. Thank you for healing me when I really needed it most.

Over To You . . .

Laura, 46

I'm 46 now, and it's really only in the last twelve years or so that I have begun to accept my body.

I grew up in the midst of 1990s heroin chic, and I have always been the antithesis of that look – five foot ten with broad shoulders and curves. Added to that, my parents were (and remain) very fatphobic. You have talked about the impact of body- and food-shaming comments from those we love, so you'll understand the destructive impact this had on my body image. I just thought that my body was wrong in every way and that I had to do everything I could to change it.

Throughout my teens and twenties, I had very disordered eating and a terrible relationship with food, constantly going from one fad or mainstream diet to another. You'll be unsurprised to hear that my weight yo-yoed massively, making me feel like a total failure. In my late twenties, I discovered exercise, but only as a way to burn more calories and rectify my 'eating mistakes'. Looking back, I don't know how I was functioning. I was miserable, and my body must have been in survival mode. No matter what I did, I hated my body because it was still never good enough.

The start of the shift was becoming a mum. I have two beautiful sons, now aged fifteen and twelve, and something clicked in my mind following both those pregnancies – being grateful to my body and realizing its power because it could create these two wonderful humans. It brought a new perspective and made me start to appreciate my body in a way that had never even occurred to me before.

I started to relax about what I was eating because I realized that what I ate was to fuel my sons as well as me. That relaxation totally shifted my mindset and interrupted my disordered thinking about food and my body. I can't tell you the calorie content of anything anymore because it doesn't matter. All that matters is 'Is it delicious?' and 'Do I want to eat it?' My food choices are now healthier, more interesting and varied because I'm no longer in a stranglehold of terror about the consequences of eating something. And I really love food, so it's wonderful to be able to enjoy it!

Another major shift over the past ten years has been my relationship with exercise. It is no longer a punishment or a control mechanism, but my primary tool for my mental health. I try and do something every morning (some days it's half an hour and some days it's literally two minutes!) and I consciously tell myself that I am doing this first and foremost for my mind. Keeping my body healthy as well is just a lovely added bonus! That small shift in perspective changed everything. I exercise to invest in me and have a positive impact on my day, not to control or punish.

Leading on from that, I wanted to mention rugby. Your ambassadorship of the Women's Rugby World Cup makes my heart sing! I don't play, but my husband and both sons do, so as a family we are really involved in our local club and watch a lot of games. Being connected to the rugby community has been so positive for my body image and similarly I hope it will also be a great asset for my sons. Rugby is a safe space for body image because it needs and celebrates every body type. No one gets turned away or shamed for their size. I am so grateful that we have incredible athletes like the Red Roses for young girls and boys to aspire to. They are the perfect example that not everyone is built to be thin,

Over To You...

but that every body type is valuable, worthy of love and capable of success! I get quite emotional when we watch or go to Red Roses games, seeing women of all shapes being celebrated – wonderful!

Body image really is a journey, isn't it, and I'm sure mine is pretty typical. Despite my progress, the next potential challenge is now looming with the menopause. I am very conscious that I have to try and keep hold of the lessons I have learned as my body changes with age. I think this is going to be hard, particularly with a mum who is still on a constant diet even in her seventies. Nevertheless, I'm determined to be grateful for a body that's brought me so much joy and success in life.

Anna, 40

I turned 40 this year, and with three daughters stepping into their teenage years, I find myself reflecting on all the work I've done within myself. Growing up in the 1990s and 2000s, when being skinny was seen as everything, left its mark on me. But I've worked hard to unlearn those messages so my girls can inherit something different – something kinder.

As a midwife, I have the privilege of seeing women in all their shapes, sizes, and strengths, and I try each day to offer them compassion and encouragement. In many ways, the work I do with women and the work I do within myself are connected, shaping the legacy I want to pass on to my daughters.

I know the future will never be perfect, and unlearning these old beliefs is an ongoing project, but I truly believe women are growing stronger every day – and that gives me so much hope for the generations to come.

Over To You . . .

Daisy, 31

I can remember exactly when I first felt uncomfortable in my body. I was only seven, already going through puberty, and I hated how big my thighs looked compared to the other children at my small rural school. By Year 5, I was in adult clothes, unable to fit into school uniform, and filled with shame I didn't know how to process. I tried to hide myself by becoming a tomboy, cutting my hair short and wearing only boys' clothes. But one of my teachers made things worse. He humiliated me by commenting on my size in front of others.

High school brought new challenges. Suddenly my body was sexualised, and not knowing how to cope, I leaned into it, becoming blonder, dressing to attract male attention. This made me a target of bullying from other girls. By the time I left high school, I was distraught and wanted to disappear.

When I started sixth form, I decided the only way forward was to shrink myself. I had ambitions of going to Oxford, so I moved to an all-girls school where the standard of beauty was extremely thin and waif-like. I began smoking instead of eating. At university, it continued. I felt that having a small appetite was praised by my peers, and my studies in zoology gave me a socially acceptable way to restrict further by becoming vegan. At my worst, I was so underweight and weak that I kept fainting during a volunteer position until my parents had to come and take me home. I remember looking into a mirror at a service station and not recognizing myself – I actually pointed out the 'awful-looking person over there' to my mum before realizing it was my own reflection. I lost my period for two years whilst I was studying, and unfortunately, this has become a huge problem later in life.

Several things helped turn this around. Becoming a personal trainer was huge. I was weighing women every day, and I realized how rare it actually is to weigh under 10 stone. I saw other trainers pushing clients into dangerous levels of restriction just to have flashy 'before and after' photos, and I recognized the harm in it. Strong women build each other up. Comparison is a learned distraction, designed to keep us focused inward. When we empower one another to take up space, we create room for the conversations and changes that truly matter. For the first time, I could see myself as 'just fine' the way I was. Even when clients made comments about my body (which still happens often), I understood that those comments were a reflection of their insecurities, not proof that there was anything wrong with me. In 2023, I completed an ultramarathon. I have truly never felt more at peace than when I was doing this – I was eating for performance and I was eating a lot! I trusted my body so much.

In the past two years, another major turning point has been my fertility journey. My husband and I have been struggling to conceive, and I was diagnosed with PCOS and endometriosis. Through treatment, I learned that PCOS can make it actively harder to stay slim, and that over-exercising can actually prevent ovulation. For the first time in my life, I had an explanation for why, despite training six to ten hours a week and dieting constantly, I could never stay thin. This knowledge has been strangely freeing: my body isn't broken, it's simply working differently, and it doesn't deserve the punishment I've been giving it for so long. Moreover, I now have the knowledge that, no matter how gut-wrenching

I find it to moderate my exercise, it is more important for me to keep my body free of stress right now than to be the smallest version of myself.

    I still have terrible days where I cannot face getting dressed. I have no idea what size I am and the reflection in the mirror seems to shapeshift continually. However, going through this fertility journey is really showing me that I must have healed massively. The old me would never have prioritized a potential life above my desire to get skinny, and I am ashamed of that.

Harri, 32

Well, my body image story isn't over, so to speak. In fact, it's very much an ongoing battle. I have had an eating disorder on and off for fourteen years, and body dysmorphia has been a big part of it. But the hardest parts are also being non-binary and having lipoedema.

Lipoedema is essentially a fat storage condition affecting as many as one in ten AFAB [assigned female at birth] people. It's a progressive condition where an abnormal type of fatty tissue is deposited mainly on the legs from the hips to the ankles with sparing of the feet, creating a sort of bracelet or cuff at the ankle. Some people, me included, also have it in their arms. This leaves people with a disproportionately smaller upper body. It's a hereditary condition and is progressive, so the affected limbs will continue to grow and grow. My grannie also had lipoedema and when she died, her upper body was tiny, but her legs were so big she couldn't have a standard-size coffin. Lipoedema is resistant to diet and exercise – it cannot be lost. This has recently been shown with people with lipoedema using GLP-1s, losing large amounts of weight from their upper body but their legs and other affected areas staying the same. The only way to get rid of the tissue is a very specific form of liposuction.

Back to me! I was obese as a child (99th centile for weight and 25th for height at age 11) and continued to be overweight into my teens. Then during my sixth form years, I went to an all-girls grammar school. All the girls who were successful and high-achieving were thin. And so my logic was that if I wanted to be high-achieving and successful, I needed to be thin too. The

Over To You . . .

weight loss began. I shan't go into the details, but no matter what my weight was doing, I never seemed to get any smaller. I would look in the mirror, and my body would morph before my eyes, expanding more and more. The same happened if I ever looked at a photo. It still does now.

I think a big part of it, especially with lipoedema, is the feeling of a lack of control. Knowing that there are parts of my body I cannot change without surgery feels so incredibly unfair. I have been lucky enough to have some of the lipoedema removed, but it didn't really impact my body image as much as I thought it would. I try my best to think of my body for the things it lets me do – running, cycling, climbing mountains – tell myself that having a functioning body gives me the freedom many others don't have, but it's hard.

My gender identity has also played a big part in my body image. I am non-binary (AFAB) and when it comes to my identity, I feel very neutral. I don't feel feminine at all, really, but I also don't feel masculine. I went through female puberty and still have a female body, which makes me feel extremely dysphoric. When I am smaller, my chest is smaller, so I am much more androgynous, and feel a little more at ease for a time. Again, when I was smaller, I lost my period for a while, which also made me feel less dysphoric. So I have this strange toss-up between having a healthy body and having a body I am more comfortable in. And I think they are mutually exclusive. I guess this goes to show that there are so many factors that impact body image.

Freya, 37

I have always been the classic tall blonde girl, always very slim. When I fell pregnant with my first baby, I was a little worried about how I would look, but once my son was born, I had such a focus on him, I didn't care. Truth was, apart from a little extra tummy, I was pretty much the same. I then had two miscarriages, both during Covid. I felt like my body was failing me. The one thing we are meant to do as women is to have kids, right? And my body couldn't do it. I just felt a complete disconnect with my body.

In 2021 I had my daughter. Again, I did worry about the fact I definitely had a 'mum tum' (I really hate that phrase) but I had a daughter now. I had grown up watching my mum be self-critical and hate her body, and it made me so sad that she couldn't see what an amazing woman she is. I decided in those first newborn days to connect back to my body, to consciously talk about it kindly and be proud of all it had survived and the two amazing babies it grew and delivered. I want my daughter to know imperfections are OK in life, but our bodies are powerhouses and are what help to make us wonderful. I don't want her to ever hate her body – she is perfect to me!

Last May I discovered a tiny divot in my left breast, about half the size of my pinky nail. It hadn't been there when I did my self-check the month before. I called the GP and was seen three days later and referred to our local breast clinic. I had only finished breastfeeding three months prior, so was assured it was most likely related to that. I was seen at our local hospital within two weeks. The consultant shared the view of the GP but gave me an ultrasound anyway to be sure. Again, he was pretty certain that the changes were consistent with finishing breastfeeding, but I have health anxiety and pleaded for a mammogram. He agreed, and that was when they discovered my tumour. They took biopsies but told me they were 99 per cent sure it would come back as cancer. Right enough, five days later I got a call to come in. It was a 9.5 cm breast tumour. I was being sent to genetics for testing and also the plastic surgery team.

The plastic surgeon I was under is the most wonderful woman I have ever met. So kind, so understanding, incredible at her job, and just oozed confidence. She told me my best option for reconstruction was a DIEP, which involved removing the skin and fat from my abdomen, hip to hip, and using that to rebuild my breast once the breast surgeon had done a mastectomy. I went for that option after a lot of talks with various people and lots of research. I had my twelve-and-a-half-hour surgery in September and, although my recovery was textbook, it was painful and took time. I then had to have a lymph node clearance two months later.

Sadly, in December I then was told I would be starting chemo and then radiotherapy, and then ovary suppression meds and preventative treatment. Chemo has always been my biggest fear, and it proved worse than I had ever imagined. It nearly killed me twice. I lost my beautiful, very long, straight, very blonde hair. I used the cold cap, so I retained about 20 per cent of it, but the morning it started coming out was heartbreaking and is up there as one of the most traumatic moments in my life. I lost my eyelashes and eyebrows too, and I love having my lashes done – eleven years of Russian lashes! My body has been affected by the radiotherapy with some skin colour changes, and the ovary suppression means that, at thirty-seven, I am in the menopause, so I've gained a bit of weight through treatment.

Right now, I am cancer-free, but there's a high chance it will come back. It has completely ravaged my body and left me feeling betrayed and disconnected again. I have a 21 in. scar on my abdomen, a scar around my belly button, a scar on my breast like a magnifying glass, and then one in my armpit along with one on my upper arm from my chemo IV line. My hair has grown in blonde and straight just as it was, but it's a very short pixie style and I just don't look like me.

I was saying this to my plastic surgeon, and that wonderful woman changed my world. She asked me, 'Why did you fight this?' The answer was obvious – I've done it all for my kids. And she told me, 'Your kids saved your life. That skin and fat we took to rebuild you? Your babies, just by being alive and growing, they prepped that skin perfectly for me to use. That excess was there to take and to save your life. Women's bodies change forever after babies, partly for self-preservation. If you ever need a skin graft or plastic surgery, it's there to use. It's a level of protection that no other mammal on earth has.'

That one conversation has helped shift my view. My daughter is four now, and she asked about my scars the other month. I said to her that they were a good thing, a sign doctors had done their job and the badness was gone. That I was healing. Every night she now helps me to moisturise my scars. The funny thing is that my dad had cancer at my age, and I grew up so scared and sad about his scars. I hope that by showing my kids my scars, and by showing them I'm trying to take care of them and love them, that my children will grow up knowing how incredible our bodies are, but also without the fear I had.

I grew up through all the 'skinny is best', 'look who's got fat' (shocker – they were never fat!). I share a lot of the body hang-ups of other women my age, but I am working so hard to appreciate all my body has been through, all it has given me, and to protect it as much as I can. I just want to make sure I'm around to see the wonderful people I know my children will grow up to become.

Would I love to be the size 8, anxiety-free girl I was at 21? Yes, I would, but today, typing this with the sound of my kids snoring, tucked up safely in bed, and sitting next to a husband who adores me and who I adore back, I wouldn't change any of it. If anything, I'm more determined to get women talking about their bodies and self-checking regularly!

Conclusion

Every person whose story you read here – including mine – has wrestled with shame, expectation, comparison, sometimes with illness and loss. Each one of us has found, in our own way, something to hold on to despite the pain – whether it's joy in wearing shorts to the beach, the pride of nourishing a child, or the act of softening towards scars.

None of us chose the culture we were born into; the beauty ideals we were handed; or the judgements that were waiting for us before our bodies had even stopped maturing. But together, we are choosing something else! We're choosing strength and resilience and rebellion and resolving to make a better world. For our children, yes, but also for the women who came before us and the ones who will come after. Most crucially of all, we're doing it for ourselves. These stories – our stories – are proof of that.

As I close this book, I want to make sure the conversation is kept open. We are never alone – and every time one of us speaks honestly about how we feel about our bodies, we not only open the door for connection and healing, we create space for someone else to share their own story.

The future is louder, braver . . . and it belongs to *all* of us.

Acknowledgements

Writing this book took place alongside some of the most transformative and emotionally challenging months of my life.
It began in the tender, disorienting period after becoming a mother for the first time and continued into the physical and emotional intensity of IVF. There were days when the writing flowed easily and days when it required patience, negotiation and a willingness to keep going in smaller increments. This book was written inside that reality, and, in many ways, because of it.

For that, I need to thank everyone whose patience, flexibility and trust allowed this book the time and space it needed to become what it is. First things first, my brilliant editor Marleigh Price: thank you for your belief in this book from the very beginning, and for the calm, steady confidence you brought to the process. Your clarity, unwavering support and patience made it possible for me to write honestly and without compromise.

I must thank the wider publishing team at HQ, and of course the inimitable Lisa Milton. I'll never forget the moment when, after a panel at Primadonna festival (which took a few unexpected conversational turns I'm not able to repeat here) Lisa turned to me, completely casually, and said 'So . . . we're doing book two, yeah?'

The words rang in my ears as I left, one of those rare, pinch-me moments. I turned to my husband, Dave, still slightly stunned, and said, 'I think I'm doing another book'. He replied, 'Of course you are,' without missing a beat.

Speaking of Dave, that quiet confidence was exactly what carried me through the writing of this book. From absorbing more than your fair share of the practical load, to keeping things steady on the days when I felt anything but, you made it possible for me to keep showing up to the page. I could not have written this book without you.

To the third person in our relationship: my sister Jen! What started as helping with bits here and there quickly became something much bigger. Somewhere along the way, you stopped being my unofficial support system and became my full-time business partner, my sounding board and the person I turn to for advice when I need clarity and honesty – the way only sisters can give it! – in equal measure. You were my rock while writing this book, and I don't take for granted for a second how lucky I am that we get to do this work together. I know you care about it as much as I do, and that means everything.

In fact, Jen and my three other wonderful sisters, Katherine, Ellie and Sophie, are the reason I care so deeply about this work. Seeing their worth so clearly, which extends far beyond appearance or performance, has made it impossible for me to accept the narrow definitions of beauty, value and success we are so often handed – definitions designed to keep women small. My relationship with my sisters keeps me grounded in purpose.

And of course, behind all of us are our very brilliant parents. To my mum and dad, Norma and David: thank you endlessly

Acknowledgements

for the unwavering support that has carried me from the very beginning. For encouraging me – even when you weren't always entirely sure what I was doing! – and for backing me without question. Your belief, generosity and constant presence have made possible more than I can ever properly put into words.

I would also love to take a moment to thank someone who has changed my life in ways I am still discovering – psychologist Dr Jude McLean. You were instrumental in helping me cultivate the self-compassion I was desperately lacking for so long, which has subsequently allowed me to unlock a much deeper compassion for others – something that has proved integral to the work I do now.

Speaking of gratitude: I would never be here without this community, without you. You have read, questioned, challenged and trusted me over the years, and your stories have sharpened my thinking, raised the stakes of this work and reminded me constantly why it matters. I don't take that lightly, and from the bottom of my heart: thank you.

And lastly, to my son, Tommy. Thank you for changing everything – my life, my mind, my heart... I am infinitely better because of you. This book is, in many ways, a response to the world I want you to grow up in: one where bodies are not measured by their appearance, and where worth is never conditional. I love you beyond measure.

Endnotes

[1] Fardouly, J., et al. (2023). 'Small exposure to body positive content can improve body image'. UNSW Sydney. School of Psychology. https://www.unsw.edu.au/newsroom/news/2023/01/small-exposure-to-body-positive-content-can-improve-body-image

[2] Rodgers, R. F., et al. (2024). 'Exposure to body-positive content improves body satisfaction and reduces drive for thinness: An experimental study'. *Appetite*, 195, 107065. https://doi.org/10.1016/j.bodyim.2024.101841

[3] Homan, K. J. & Tylka, T. L. (2020). 'Exposure to body diversity images as a buffer against the thin-ideal: An experimental study'. *Body Image*, 33, 270–279. https://doi.org/10.1016/j.bodyim.2020.03.007

[4] Figueroa, E. (2023). 'Reality TV lacks body diversity - and it matters for viewers' self-esteem'. *Verywell Mind*. https://www.verywellmind.com/reality-tv-lacks-body-diversity-8748350

[5] *Hopkins Medicine Newsroom*. (2024, December). 'Eating Disorders Among Kids Are on the Rise'. https://www.hopkinsmedicine.org/news/articles/2024/12/eating-disorders-among-kids-are-on-the-rise

[6] *Financial Times*. (2023, March). 'The Teen Mental Health Crisis: A Reckoning for Big Tech'. https://www.ft.com/content/77d06d3e-2b9f-4d46-814f-da2646fea60c

[7] Pitchforth, J., et al. (2023). 'Alarming Increase of Eating Disorders in Children and Adolescents'. *Journal of Pediatrics*, vol. 260, 2023, pp. 113–121. https://www.jpeds.com/article/S0022-3476%2823%2900596-6/fulltext

[8] Judge, T. A., Cable, D. M. (2011). 'When It Comes to Pay, Do the Thin Win? The Effect of Weight on Pay for Men and Women'. *Journal of Applied Psychology*, 96, no. 1 (2011)

[9] Cawley, John, (2004). 'The Impact of Obesity on Wages'. *Journal of Human Resources* 39, no. 2 (2004): 451–474

[10] Wilding, J. P. H., et al. (2021). 'Once-Weekly Semaglutide in Adults with Overweight or Obesity'. *New England Journal of Medicine*, 384(11): 989–1002. DOI: 10.1056/NEJMoa2032183

[11] Jastreboff, A. M., et al. (2022). 'Tirzepatide Once Weekly for the Treatment of Obesity'. *New England Journal of Medicine*, 387(3): 205–216. DOI: 10.1056/NEJMoa2206038

[12] Weight regain following the cessation of GLP-1 RAs for weight management: a systematic review and meta-analysis. Nuffield Department of Primary Care Health Sciences, University of Oxford

[13] According to analysis by Verity, an insider trading research and analytics firm

[14] City University of London. (2020). 'Changing the Perfect Picture: Smartphones, Social Media and Appearance Pressures'. https://www.citystgeorges.ac.uk/__data/assets/pdf_file/0005/597209/Parliament-Report-web.pdf

[15] Spotlight on America. (2024, March). 'Social media beauty filters impacting the mental health of young women'. The National News Desk. Retrieved from https://thenationaldesk.com/news/spotlight-on-america/social-media-beauty-filters-impacting-the-mental-health-of-young-women-tiktok-meta-snapchat-instagram-university-of-london-study-bold-glamour-facetune-bodytune-airbrush

[16] O'Doherty, J., et al. (2003). 'Beauty in a smile: The role of the medial orbitofrontal cortex in facial attractiveness'. *Neuropsychologia*, 41(2): 147–155

[17] Nightingale, S. J. & Farid, H. (2022). 'AI-synthesized faces are indistinguishable from real faces and more trustworthy'. *PNAS*, 119(8)

[18] 'Virtual Try-On Technology for the Luxury Industry: How It Works, Benefits & Challenges'. Wanna Fashion. https://wanna.fashion/blog/virtual-try-on-technology-for-luxury-industry

[19] Riccio, P., Colin, J., Ogolla, S. & Oliver, N. (2024). 'Mirror, Mirror

on the Wall, Who Is the Whitest of All? Racial Biases in Social Media Beauty Filters'. *Social Media + Society*, 10(2)

[20] Hendeniya, H. M. U. S. (2025). 'The Impact of AI Filters on Beauty Standards in Sri Lanka'

[21] Woeyram Anani, et al. (2024). 'Filtered Reality: Exploring the Motives and Socio-Demographic Factors of Smartphone Beauty Filter Usage Among University Students in Ghana'

[22] Chen, T., Lian, K., et al. (2020). 'Occidentalisation of Beauty Standards: Eurocentrism in Asia'. *Across the Spectrum of Socioeconomics*, 1(2): 1–11

[23] Mateusz Grajek, Tomasz Jurys, Mateusz Rozmiarek, (2024). 'Gender differences in digital beauty engagement.' *Cogent Psychology*, 11(1): 2392381. https://doi.org/10.1080/23311983.2024.2392381

[24] Tiggemann, M. & Anderberg, I. (2020). 'Social media is not real: The effect of 'Instagram vs reality' images on women's social comparison and body image.' *New Media & Society*, 22(12): 2183–2199. https://doi.org/10.1177/1461444819888720

[25] Fardouly, J., et al. (2018). 'Social comparisons on social media: The impact of Facebook on young women's body image concerns and mood'. *Body Image*, 13: 38–45. https://doi.org/10.1016/j.bodyim.2014.12.003

[26] McLean, S. A., et al. (2023). 'Photo-editing and self-objectification: The mediating role of appearance comparisons'. *BMC Psychology*, 11(1): 143. https://doi.org/10.1186/s40359-023-01143-0

[27] Mironica, A., Popescu, C. A., George, D., Tegzeșiu, A. M. and Gherman, C. D. (2024) 'Social media influence on body image and cosmetic surgery considerations: a systematic review', Cureus, 16(7), p. e65626. doi: 10.7759/cureus.65626

[28] Gupta, M., Jassi, A. & Krebs, G. (2023). 'The association between social media use and body dysmorphic symptoms in young people'. *Frontiers in Psychology*, 14: 1231801

[29] Buolamwini, J., Gebru, T. (2018). *Gender Shades: Intersectional Accuracy Disparities in Commercial Gender Classification.* https://proceedings.mlr.press/v81/buolamwini18a/buolamwini18a.pdf

[30] Mintel, *Colour Cosmetics Consumer Report*, 2023

31 Stonewall, *LGBT in Britain: Trans Report*, 2022

32 Johnson, S.K., et al. (2018). 'Perceptions of competence and attractiveness in the workplace'. *Journal of Applied Psychology*

33 Fortune Business Insights. (2024). 'Global cosmetics market valued at USD 335.95 billion, projected to reach USD 556.21 billion by 2032'

34 Exploding Topics. (2025, July) 'Average U.S. women spend over $10/day or ~$3,756/year on beauty products' (Groupon/OnePoll data)

35 GoBankingRates. (2023). 'How Much Gen Z, Millennial, Gen X and Boomer Women Spend on Beauty'

36 Mafra, A. L. et al. (2022). 'The contrasting effects of body image and self-esteem in the makeup usage.' PLOS ONE 17(3): e0265197

37 Arizton Advisory & Intelligence. (2024). *Color Cosmetics Market – Global Outlook & Forecast 2024–2029*. Notes the global color cosmetics market was USD 76.5 billion in 2023. Available at: https://www.arizton.com/market-reports/color-cosmetics-market

38 American Society of Plastic Surgeons. (2005). *2005 Procedural Statistics Report*

39 Fortune Business Insights. (2023). *Cosmetic Surgery and Procedure Market Size Report 2023*

40 *The Times*. (2025, July). 'Britain is obsessed with beauty procedures. These figures prove it.'

41 *InStyle*. (2022, December). 'Cosmetic Treatments Were Once Considered Taboo — Times Have Changed.'

42 American Society of Plastic Surgeons. (2015 & 2019). *Plastic Surgery Statistics Reports*

43 Save Face. (2018). *Annual Complaint Report*

44 British Association of Aesthetic Plastic Surgeons (BAAPS). (2021)

45 Grand View Research. (2023). *Anti-Aging Market Size Report*

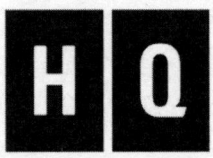

ONE PLACE. MANY STORIES

Bold, innovative and empowering publishing.

FOLLOW US ON:

@HQStories